Your Body's
Environmental
CHEMICAL
Burden

A Resource Guide
to Understanding and Avoiding Toxins

CINDY KLEMENT, *MS, CNS, MCHES*

Published by Mindstir Media, LLC
45 Lafayette Rd | Suite 181| North Hampton, NH 03862 | USA
1.800.767.0531 | www.mindstirmedia.com

Printed in the United States of America
ISBN-13: 978-1-7327049-6-1
Library of Congress Control Number: 2018911590

For Dr. Lev (Ed) Linkner,
with love and appreciation
for all you have done, and continue to do,
to support me with my health, my education,
and in my career.

For my children,
thank you for trusting me
to experiment with your health,
and your children's health, and for allowing me
into your medicine cabinets and pantries.

For my husband Michael,
with utmost gratitude
for your never-ending support,
and your constant love, encouragement, and enthusiasm,
as none of this could have been possible without you.

ENDORSEMENTS

"Your Body's Environmental Chemical Burden is a treasure trove of toxin information for the 21st century. It is the new go-to toxin reference, so you can understand what you are exposed to and how to avoid the spectrum of contaminants. Every home should have this book!"

- Deanna Minich, PhD, *author of Whole Detox: A 21-Day Personalized Program to Break Through Barriers in Every Area of Your Life*

"Cindy Klement has prepared an important and practical book that provides essential information on the issue of common environmental chemicals that are affecting the health and well-being of so many people throughout the world. By reading this well-written and powerful work, readers will acquire a good understanding of the prominence of the chemical burden challenge and be personally empowered to make a major difference in the lives of those around them."

- Stephen Genuis, *MD, FRCSC, DABOG, DABEM, FAAEM, Clinical Professor, Faculty of Medicine, University of Alberta, Edmonton, Canada*

"Eye opening information everyone should be aware of. The bad news is that our environment continues to become more and more toxic. The good news is we now have this resource to help guide us toward better and 'less toxic' living. Highly recommended!"

- Luis N. Pacheco, *MD, FAAFP, Board-Certified in Family Medicine, Clinical Associate Professor, University of Southern California Emmy-Award Winning Doctor and one of the most widely recognized physicians in the U.S. Latino community*

CONTENTS

PREFACE

In the fall of 2013 I attended a lecture on health. The presenter at the time used the term 'body burden.' I assumed that the burden he spoke of was that which most of us carry, meaning either our emotional burden or the burden of excess body weight. The term stuck with me for a very long time, piquing my curiosity. As a professor I have access to thousands of peer-reviewed scientific journals through the university online library, so one day I decided to see if searching 'body burden' would yield any published research. Much to my surprise over 420,000 journal articles were immediately at my fingertips and as I narrowed the search to only the previous three years, the database still revealed over 123,000 results.

As I scrolled down through the selection I began to note that many of the articles were from prestigious journals such as *Food Additives & Contaminants*, *Environmental Pollution*, *Environmental Health*

Perspectives, and *Environmental Toxicology and Chemistry,* among so many others. After downloading and reading several of the studies I began to realize the term had more to do with the body's environmental chemical burden than the emotional or weight burden.

The more I downloaded and read, the more alarmed I became and wanted to know which chemicals might be lurking silently in my body's tissues. I questioned whether or not there may indeed be some stored toxicant that could explain the idiopathic vertigo I had dealt with for almost sixty years, and as I learned more and more about the effects chemicals can have on our overall health I became consumed with study.

Results of My Toxicology Testing

In March of 2014 I asked my dear friend and personal physician Dr. Lev (Ed) Linkner if we could run a toxicant profile using blood and urine. He told me to find the test I'd like to have and he'd be glad to order it. Genova Diagnostics offered a quite pricey Toxic Effects Profile that tested for 45 chemicals found in humans, including volatile organic compounds (VOCs), chlorinated and organophosphate pesticides, PCBs, BPA, phthalates, and parabens.

For a woman of 63 years at the time who had been eating virtually organic since the late 1970s and used the safest personal care and cleaning products for almost four decades, it came as a complete surprise when the results showed I was in the 80th percentile for benzene and styrene, the 95th percentile for PCB153, and had detectable levels of DDE, phthalates, pesticides, BPA, and parabens. Being in the 95th percentile means only 5% of other individuals that were tested exceeded the level found in my body. I am not a chemist by any stretch of the imagination so I had absolutely no idea what these chemicals were, how they got into my tissue, or if I could ever get them out.

Research Commences

I could not stop researching these chemical contaminants whenever I found extra time. From March of 2014 until the end of the year, I accumulated over 1,500 studies on the topic of the body's environmental chemical burden. I read each one of them (mostly on airplanes and in hotel rooms) and highlighted notes I felt were pertinent. I learned what the chemicals are used for, and how many millions (and sometimes billions or trillions) of pounds are produced around the world. I came to understand how we are exposed and the health effects that can occur both in humans and in the animal kingdom. And with each new chemical I became increasingly concerned about the future of our children and their children. I especially became concerned for the millennial generation and the hardships they will face as a result of the worldwide environmental chemical contamination.

"Healthy" Products

While writing this book I had to examine my own lifestyle and was able to make even more changes than I ever knew I needed to. Things as simple as changing the cutting boards in the kitchen, throwing out the hair dryer and air popcorn maker from the 1970s, getting better skin care products and shampoos even though what I was using was considered organic. I learned that recycled paper contains more BPA than virgin paper, which presents a dilemma. I've always tried to take care of my planet by recycling and using recycled products. Now I'm in a quandary over whether or not to continue using toilet paper and paper towels from recycled paper.

I was already aware of healthier cleaning products, although when I first began using them in the late 1970s they left much to be desired. They simply didn't clean things well enough. It wasn't until a few years ago when one of the companies I teach for added healthy cleaning products to their growing product line. I was to lecture across the U.S. on the efficacy of these products so I wanted to make sure they worked before I touted their benefits. One product, in particular, got my attention. It was a laundry powder used to whiten clothing. I never use chlorinated bleach products to clean my sinks and tubs and toilets because the odor bothers my respiratory system, resulting in porcelain and tile that never appeared to be quite clean. Curious, I wondered if this laundry powder would also whiten the tub. Much to my surprise it did, with no odor or toxic chemicals. Today I use either BioKleen's powder or the 365 brand from Whole Foods.

My Personal Dilemma

I still cook a homemade organic meal almost every night and sit down with my husband at the dinner table. As my research continued I realized that organic wasn't always the best, depending on where the food was grown and how it was processed. I started to question other foods in our diet when data revealed fish was toxic and so were some legumes and leafy greens. Dairy products could also be problematic... and the list went on and on. I became more and more concerned about what to prepare for our meals. During dinner, the conversation would inevitably turn to what I'd learned during that particular day's studies, and the discussions became more and more sobering over the months that followed. In fact, so much so that I needed to take a break from study and think about what I was going to do with this newfound knowledge. Would anyone be interested in learning about this vast topic?

Can My Research Help Others?

I have maintained a private practice in integrative and functional health since 1983. So when I met with clients I began to ask them about their physical environment after they shared their health concerns. The story of one such family comes to mind. A young Korean couple came to see me for feelings of rawness in their throats and bronchial tubes, as all their medical tests came back normal and the medication they were prescribed did nothing to alleviate the discomfort. So I asked about their occupations, their commutes, where they lived, what they ate and drank, any recent remodeling, and finally about their cleaning products. Interestingly, each night after cleaning up the dinner meal this couple would use chlorine bleach to sanitize the counter top! Had no one ever thought to ask about their cleaning practices? Apparently not. Within weeks of eliminating the use of bleach the couple no longer experienced their throat issues. Another time, switching laundry detergent and eliminating dryer sheets used on the baby's clothing, sheets, and towels helped heal a young infant of her eczema.

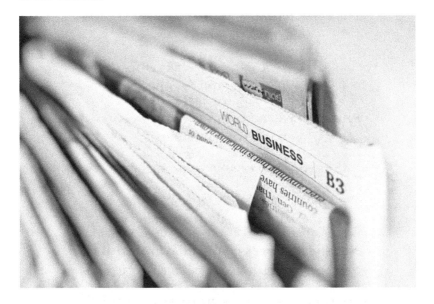

In the News

Was I onto something here? Headline after headline began catching my attention, including the following:

- EPA: POLLUTION FROM MINE SPILL
  MUCH WORSE THAN FEARED

- COULD POLLUTION BE TO BLAME FOR WHY
  DEMENTIA IS KILLING MORE PEOPLE?

- THE MOST POLLUTED CITIES IN AMERICA

- LITTLE KIDS GETTING DRUNK
  ON FRUITY HAND SANITIZERS

- USE TOOTHPASTE AND FACE WASH WITH MICROBEADS?
  STOP NOW

- FAMILY SUES TERMINEX;
  SON UNABLE TO WALK AFTER FUMIGATION

- MORE EVIDENCE CHILDREN HARMED BY LEAD NEAR
  PHILADELPHIA 'GHOST FACTORY'

- FORD PLANT'S TOXIC GROUNDWATER PLUME CREEPING
  TOWARD NEIGHBORHOOD

- UNHEALTHY ENVIRONMENT A FACTOR IN MILLIONS
  OF DEATHS WORLDWIDE

- IS YOUR WATER SAFE FROM DIOXANE?

- MICHIGAN REJECTS PLAN TO DEREGULATE
  HUGE LIST OF TOXIC AIR CHEMICALS

- WATER STREET PCB CONTAMINATION PROMPTS
  YPSILANTI TO CLOSE BORDER TO BORDER TRAIL

- REPORT CLAIMS DIOXANE PLUME POSES IMMINENT
  PUBLIC HEALTH RISK IN ANN ARBOR

- EPA CONCERNED ABOUT URGENT" SITUATION
  WITH CHLORINE LEVELS IN FLINT WATER

- UNKNOWNS DRIVE TOXIC WATER WORRIES NEAR
  OLD MICHIGAN AIR FORCE BASE

- TRAIN CARRYING OIL DERAILS,
  BURNS IN COLUMBIA GORGE

- UM STUDY: PESTICIDE EXPOSURE
  MAY BE ALS RISK FACTOR

- VETERANS BLAME AIR FORCE BASE WATER
  FOR CHRONIC DISEASES

- JURORS: DUPONT ACTED WITH MALICE;
  $5M DUE TO MAN WITH CANCER

- U.S. STEEL LAWSUIT STALLS DETROIT
  AIR POLLUTION PLAN

- $1M FINE FOR SHIP THAT DUMPED OILY WATER IN
  GREAT LAKES AND TRIED TO HIDE IT

- 'ERIN BROCKOVICH' TOXIN FOUND IN DRINKING WATER

It's Time

I decided it was time to share the information I'd uncovered with other people, however, I'd never written a book before. Sure, I've written two theses but never a book and I had absolutely no idea how to go about organizing the notes from my 1,500+ studies. Also, the story wasn't pretty and I was concerned readers may feel as overwhelmed and helpless as I did when I first began to understand the pervasive effects of environmental chemicals. After much contemplation, in January of 2015, I simply decided to open a new Word document and begin to tell the story, one chemical at a time.

I wanted to share with others how I would avoid future chemical contamination of the chemicals found in my body and decided that each chapter would host a resource section to provide the tools necessary for readers to examine possible exposures occurring through their occupations, their commutes, their arts and crafts supplies, personal care products, foods, cleaning supplies, clothing, and dishware, among others. I also wanted to share how to get these chemicals out of the body whenever possible. Yet I found research on detoxification quite scarce.

Sifting through the Research

As I mentioned above, I was able to locate over 123,000 studies published in a three-year period on our exposure to toxicants, and yet very few researchers have focused on how to eliminate them from our bodies. The final chapter in this book, Detoxification, would not be possible without the work of Dr. Stephen J. Genuis from the University of Alberta, Edmonton, and Margaret E. Sears at Children's Hospital of Eastern Ontario Research Institute in Ottawa, Canada. Their contribution to the field of environmental medicine and human detoxification is extraordinary and readers will find much of their work referenced throughout this entire guide.

While writing this book I began to lecture on the topic across the U.S. and Canada, and people have shown a tremendous interest in this topic. The point I make during my lectures is this: chemicals are here to stay and we have to learn to co-exist with them. We can't avoid every one of them, but we can use the tools and resources at our disposal to reduce our exposure. We can also detoxify the body as best we can with what we know now.

My Sincere Hope for Future Generations

My hope is that every one of our young millennials will get their bodies and homes as cleared of chemicals as possible before bringing children into this incredibly polluted world. It's important for them to detoxify their own bodies as much as possible so the sperm is vital and healthy, and so females have fewer contaminants to pass on to their infants through the placenta and through breast milk – something readers will learn all about as they review this text.

Everyone needs to be aware of what they can and can't do to avoid adding to the body's environmental chemical burden, especially those contemplating future parenthood. I sincerely hope this work helps guide you to the best health possible for yourself, your children, grand-children, and great-grandchildren.

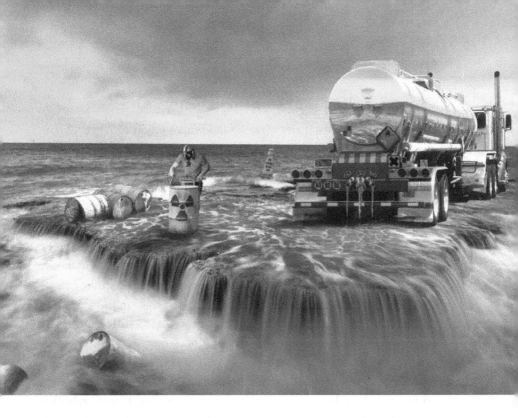

INTRODUCTION

In most medical training today there is a lack of information in the curriculum regarding environmental medicine and yet in the United States alone it is estimated that 13% of disease is attributed to the environment, amounting to almost 400,000 deaths per year from cardiovascular disease, neuropsychiatric disorders, and cancer. Exposure to environmental chemicals is rarely even mentioned in initiatives to combat chronic diseases. Distinguished Professor Emerita at University of California Davis, Judith S. Stern, stated "our genetics may load the gun, but our environment pulls the trigger." Health care systems are not trained to address the contribution of environmental contaminants and their effects on the health of the human body. Many clinicians are not yet even aware of the science behind toxicant bioaccumulation and related health consequences, nor how or where their patients are exposed.

Concerns Regarding Bioaccumulation

Sparse literature on the topic of the body's environmental chemical burden promotes controversy and ongoing debates while new chemicals are introduced without first being fully tested for toxicity, only to be taken off the market when harmful effects are proven. A lack of evidence should not be used to verify safety when no one has ever established a chemical as harmless.

Bioaccumulation (slow concentrating of chemicals in the body) of chronic low-level exposure from multiple chemical sources makes it difficult to demonstrate cause and effect because most studies focus on a single chemical, although we are rarely exposed to just one contaminant. Concerns are mounting that exposure to different classes of chemicals and their breakdown products may actually enhance toxicity and intensify their effects. Different chemicals have different health outcomes and continuous exposure to a multitude of chemical types on a daily basis results in a slurry of chemicals with additive and/or synergistic effects in the body. The key challenge in research is to determine widespread exposure to multiple sources, multiple chemical classes, varying concentrations, and the overall health of the individual.

Ethical Issues

It is not ethically possible to expose study participants to potentially dangerous exposures of environmental chemicals. Of the 85,0000 synthetic chemicals manufactured over the past four decades, little toxicity information exists. In 1976, over 60,000 chemicals were grandfathered in when the United States Congress passed the Toxic Substances Control Act. As of 2010, 17,000 chemicals under the exemption are still in use and remain available to manufacturers, some of which have questionable safety ratings.

Restricting Harmful Chemicals

The Stockholm Convention on Persistent Organic Pollutants aims to restrict or eliminate the use and production of 23 classes of chemicals. A use reduction policy in the United States has been met with political resistance, due to debates concerning the impact of policies on food processors and farmers, and on the price of food.

In 2012 the United Nations Environment Programme and the World Health Organization updated their 2002 document *State of the Science of Endocrine Disrupting Chemicals* to list key concerns for decision makers concerned about the health of humans and wildlife, indicating that the vast majority of chemicals have never been tested and that this lack of data establishes significant uncertainties about the factual and accurate extent of risks that could disrupt the endocrine system. The document states that up to 40% of men in certain countries have low semen quality; that penile malformations have increased over time in baby boys, as have non-descending testes. Prostate and testicular cancer have been increasing over the past 50 years and type 2 diabetes increased from 153 million to 347 million during the past 28 years. Females are experiencing more diseases involving the breasts, ovaries, endometrium, and thyroid gland.

In 2013 the National Toxicology Program found that persistent organic pollutants, bisphenol A and phthalates, among other chemicals, were associated with diabetes and obesity in some of the populations studied. The World Health Organizations' International Programme on Chemical Safety listed 800 chemicals capable of interfering with hormone receptors, again acknowledging that the vast majority of chemicals have not been tested.

COMPLICATIONS IN RESEARCH

Why one person might react to a specific contaminant and another does not has a great deal to do with multiple factors including age, nutritional status, overall health, genetic makeup, dietary and exercise habits, functioning of detoxification systems and the chemical's target organs, as well as the developmental stages at the time of exposure, and the level and frequency of exposure.

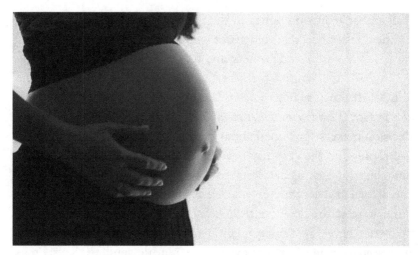

Prenatal and Early Life Exposure

Once regarded as protective, research has firmly established that the placental barrier does not shield the unborn from toxicant exposure. Over ten years ago studies determined that newborn cord blood contained an average of 287 toxicants. Breast milk and meconium studies have also revealed the passage of toxic chemicals to developing infants. Unfortunately, a number of these toxic compounds have long induction periods (the amount of time it takes to produce ill effects) so their impact won't be realized for many years. Because many of the chemicals resist elimination and persist in human tissue, there is an enormous potential to disrupt physiological processes. The Pediatric Academic Societies affirmed that the functioning of the current generation may be impacted by low level exposure to environmental chemical toxicity. Some changes may extend for generations beyond that initially exposed, a type of effect known as epigenetic.

The Human Early Life Exposome Project is researching early life exposure that begins prenatally and continues through developing years. Contact to flame retardants on bedding and sleepwear; bathing in or drinking chlorinated water; the use of personal care products; breathing vehicle exhaust or chemical air-fresheners; exposure to off-gassing in building materials inside the home or child care center; plastic bottles, utensils, and dishware; pesticides, artificial colors, flavors and preservatives in foods; house cleaning products and disinfectants, all add to the body burden of children. The project's goal is to better understand how chemical exposures influence the risk of disease.

How to Use This Book

This book details what is currently known about the most common chemical contaminants in our environment and is designed to educate readers on where they are stored, what they are used for, where and how we get exposed, and how they enter our body and affect our health. Readers can determine from a list of occupations whether exposure is likely to occur at work and the steps to be taken to ensure limited exposure. Lists are also available for personal exposure and exposure in the home. Included with each contaminant is a list of associated health concerns. At the end of each chapter a Resources and Suggestions area lists a tremendous array of useful tools, links, and sound advice on how to limit exposure whenever possible. Included in the resources is the section "Empower Yourself with These Action Steps," which is a step-by-step arsenal of tips to reinforce your protection against contaminants. For a complete list of all the resource links provided in this book see the Appendix, and to help with terminology that might not be familiar a Glossary has also been provided.

The final chapter of this text is on Detoxification. Please note, no action should be taken based solely on this book's content regardless of the perceived scientific merit. Instead readers should consult health care professionals on any matter related to their health. The information in this text is not to be considered as offering medical advice, although it may provide a clue as to some of the unresolved medical issues one might be experiencing. The content of this book is taken from recent peer-reviewed, published scientific studies and is provided for informational purposes only. It should not be used as a substitute for medically supervised therapy, as one should never disregard medical advice or delay in seeking it because of something read, especially in the field of medicine where information changes rapidly. If you suspect that you suffer from nutritional deficiencies, consult a licensed, qualified physician.

Locating a Physician Trained in Environmental Medicine

On the American College of Occupational and Environmental Medicine website readers can search by zip code for a physician specializing in environmental health. The website is available at: **https://www.acoem.org/DoctorFinderSearch.aspx**. On the American Academy of Environmental Medicine website readers can search by state for a physician. The website is available at: **https://www.aaemonline.org/**. University hospitals also have clinicians specializing in occupational and environmental medicine. To locate, enter the university name along with environmental medicine into the search bar, for example "Yale Environmental Medicine."

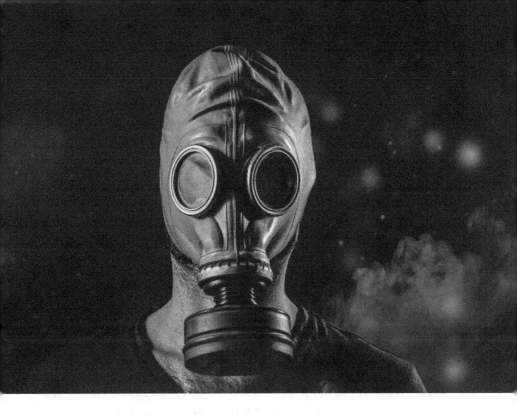

Chapter 1
TOXIC GASES:
Volatile Organic Compounds – VOCs

Of the ten most common VOCs regulated by the United States Environmental Protection Agency, five (benzene, toluene, ethylbenzene, xylene, and styrene) are in a family of compounds to which most of the population is regularly exposed through a wide array of sources. VOCs are emitted into the air during industrial processing, fuel exhaust, solvent use, and from landfills and waste treatment plants. Studies report that people spend 80-93% of their lives indoors, 2-7% outdoors, and 1-7% in an enclosed motor vehicle.

Along with contamination from outside sources, smoke from cigarettes and the burning of incense, building and renovation materials, furniture, cleaning supplies, and air fresheners contribute to concentrations inside the building. As people spend a significant amount of time in the home, exposures can occur domestically. VOC concentrations can increase dramatically during the refueling of motor vehicles and during high traffic exhaust. Each year over two million military and commercial workers are exposed to aviation fuel containing benzene, toluene, ethylbenzene, and xylene. VOC chemicals are widely used in a large number of household products including detergents, solvents, cleaning products, waxes, paints, and varnishes. Indoor air is contaminated by the same sources as outside air by both seepages into building structures and by opening windows where concentrations may be higher.

Printers and Copiers

It has been shown that these chemicals are also emitted while personal home copiers and printers are in use. When heat occurs as part of the printing process to bond toner particles to paper, residues are released and emitted from materials. A 2012 study was conducted to evaluate the effect laser printer emissions have on lung cells. Results showed that even in standby mode both particulate matter and VOCs were emitted into the air suggesting that photocopiers, fax machines, and laser printers should be completely turned off when not in use. One-third of the 62 models tested emitted ultra-fine particles in high levels, small enough to enter even the tiniest air passageways and perhaps adding to health concerns of the respiratory, immune, and nervous systems. Previous studies found copy workers to have an increase in immune system disorders.

Fragrances

Artificial fragrances added to household products can contain upwards of several hundred chemicals, some of which are classified as hazardous or toxic under Federal ruling. The results of a study on common fragranced laundry detergent and dryer sheets showed that more than 25 VOCs were emitted from dryer vents, two of which are classified by the EPA as carcinogenic (cancer causing) and seven as hazardous. Interestingly, none of the VOCs were listed on the Material Safety Data Sheet (MSDS) or product label, as labeling ingredients in household products is not required. Thus the consumer knows little about the potential for toxicant exposure while cleaning or doing laundry, where emissions from chemicals are mixed into the air and inhaled by occupants.

Bottled Water

Traces of VOC compounds can leach from plastic drinking bottles into water, especially under high temperatures and humidity, causing adverse effects on human health. The VOC concentration in bottled water increases with exposure to UV light and with storage time. Researchers found that after 5 months of storage in sunlight concentrations of xylene and ethylbenzene were increased, and toluene was found in every sample regardless of whether it was stored at room temperature or in direct sunlight.

Noted Health Effects

VOCs are associated with numerous disorders in the body. Several of these components can even react with DNA. The short-term effects can include headaches, dizziness, memory impairment, irritation of the eyes and respiratory tract, and visual disorders. Long-term exposure can result in damage to the central nervous system, the kidneys, and the liver. These solvents can also cause sleep disturbances and neuropsychiatric symptoms. Many studies report a significantly increased risk of suicide and depression from low to moderate levels of exposure to VOCs.

Results of research also show a correlation between VOC exposure and cardiovascular, visual, and auditory complications. Additionally, some research suggests high levels of occupational exposure to VOCs can affect blood pressure. Styrene has been associated with coronary artery disease, while benzene and xylene have been linked to arterial hypertension. Xylene levels increase in those with more adipose tissue. The association between chemicals and related health effects becomes problematic when individuals are exposed to varying concentrations and mixtures over time. For example, the clearance of xylene and ethylbenzene will take longer when toluene is present in the blood, and high concentrations of ethylbenzene can contribute to multiple chemical sensitivities in susceptible people.

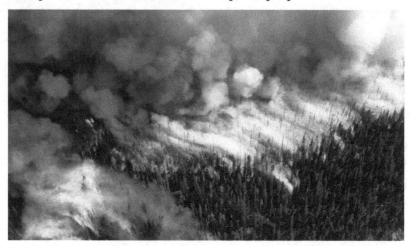

VOLATILE SOLVENTS: BENZENE

Benzene is generated as a by-product from the chemical manufacturing of petroleum-based raw materials. It belongs to a group of volatile organic compounds known as BTEXS (benzene, toluene, ethylbenzene, xylene, and styrene), accounting for roughly 60% of the chemical compounds found in large urban areas. In the United States, benzene ranks as one of the 20 most widely used chemicals. Benzene is also formed from natural processes, such as forest fires and volcanoes. Benzene exposure occurs mostly through inhalation, but can also occur through ingestion of contaminated food or water, and through skin contact. First isolated from coal tar in the 1800s, benzene is used in industry to make other chemicals. It's used in the manufacturing of pesticides, dyes, detergents, rubber, drugs, lubricants, Styrofoam, plastics, and synthetic fibers.

Environmental Exposure

Living in close proximity to petroleum manufacturing facilities and gas stations can contaminate well water with benzene when leakage occurs from underground storage tanks and hazardous waste landfills. When seepage occurs, benzene can migrate through soil and the foundation of buildings that are positioned above contaminated groundwater. Exposure then results by breathing benzene while washing dishes, doing laundry, bathing, or cooking with the contaminated water. A 2007 study indicated that people living near fueling stations that do not use a vapor-recovery system at the pump have a 3% – 21% increased risk of developing cancer of the lungs, bladder, and leucocythemia (an increased number of white blood cells in the bloodstream.) The rubber boot at the end of the fuel pump nozzle that fits directly over the gas tank opening indicates the presence of a vapor-recovery system.

Cigarettes

Benzene is one of the more dominant toxins in cigarette smoke and is associated with an increased risk of leukemia. The exposure to benzene from smoking one pack of cigarettes daily is 10 times that of a nonsmoker and levels of benzene are 30-50% higher in smokers' homes than in nonsmokers' homes. Secondhand smoke is another important source of exposure to benzene.

Indoor Air Exposure

Indoor levels often exceed outdoor levels by as much as 2 to 100 times, and are dependent on the concentration and extent of ventilation. Indoor exposure can occur from breathing the vapors from products that contain benzene, such as paint, thinners and varnish, glue and adhesives, detergent, air fresheners, moth balls, furniture wax, nail polish and hair dyes, marking pens, and art supplies.

Personal exposure may also be affected by burning wood in a wood stove, and gas heating and cooking, while automobile combustion and emissions can migrate into homes from attached garages. Burning candles in the home can increase benzene concentrations by 12%, depending on the type of candle used. Charcoal and cigarette lighting fluids additionally contribute.

Dietary Exposure

During a five-year study by the United States Food and Drug Administration, nearly every food analyzed contained benzene. Food processed at high temperatures or by irradiation have been linked to benzene, as have aromas. Currently, there are no legal limits for benzene in beverages or food. Benzene is absorbed 100% when ingested, and approximately 50% when inhaled.

Prenatal and Early Life Exposure

Benzene can pass from the mother to the fetus. In human studies, benzene has been detected in cord blood and breast milk, and is found to cause an increased incidence of premature birth. Children are also affected by benzene, and exposure has been associated with wheezing, asthma, and bronchitis.

Safety Classification

The National Toxicology Program, the United States Environmental Protection Agency, the International Agency for Research on Cancer, the Centers for Disease Control, the Agency for Toxic Substances and Disease Registry and the American Conference of Governmental Industrial Hygienists all classify benzene as a known human carcinogen. Categorized as a carcinogen, there may be no acceptable level of exposure. Currently, there is no evidence of an upper limit of exposure for its toxic effects.

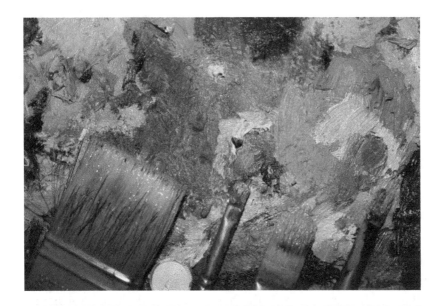

VOLATILE SOLVENTS: ETHYLBENZENE

Ethylbenzene is used primarily in styrene production and in the plastics and rubber industry, while the remainder is used as an additive in fuel, as a component of asphalt and solvents, and in the manufacture of varnish, paints, and other surface coatings. Ethylbenzene is ranked as one of the top 50 chemicals produced in the United States. Nearly 15.8 billion pounds are produced annually in Texas and Louisiana.

Ethylbenzene is absorbed in the gastrointestinal tract, through the lungs, and by the skin. The half-life of ethylbenzene is ½ to 4 hours, and it is released slowly from fat in 20-48 hours. It is secreted from the body predominantly in the urine, while the lungs and feces will also secrete small amounts.

SAFETY CLASSIFICATION

The International Agency for Research on Cancer, a subgroup of the World Health Organization, has determined that long-term exposure may cause cancer.

VOLATILE SOLVENTS: STYRENE

Styrene is used in the manufacturing of rubber, plastics, foams, resins, and fiberglass. The United States Food and Drug Administration permits styrene to be used as an additive for flavoring in foods and to make dental fillings. In 2008, 12.2 billion pounds of styrene were produced in the United States primarily in Texas and Louisiana. It has been detected in drinking water, and even in the air of an Alabama national forest.

HUMAN EXPOSURE

Styrene enters the body through inhalation, ingestion, and absorption through the skin. Once absorbed in the body, styrene circulates throughout the system with the highest levels being deposited in fat. The half-life of styrene in the human body is ½ hour to 4 hours, followed by a second phase of 13 to 30 hours. The lungs and feces can release small amounts of styrene from the body. Nursing infants can be exposed to styrene through breast milk.

DIETARY EXPOSURE

There are tremendous consumer advantages to plastics in that they are lightweight, economical, and easily stored. The concern is that styrene can migrate from packaging into food from sources such as containers with a #6 recycling code, Teflon, plastic or foam egg cartons, disposable cups and plates, carry out containers, and Styrofoam trays used in meatpacking. This is especially true when hot food and beverages are placed in Styrofoam, or microwaved in containers made with styrene, as migration increases with temperature. Due to the polystyrene containers used for milk and yogurt products, styrene has been found at higher concentrations that continue to increase during storage. However, emissions from motor vehicle exhaust and cigarette smoking are the main sources of human exposure, when not occupationally exposed.

The International Agency for Research on Cancer classifies styrene as a known mutagen (something that causes genetic mutation) and possible human carcinogen. It is classified as reasonably anticipated to be a human carcinogen by The Agency for Toxic Substances and Disease Registry and the National Toxicology Program.

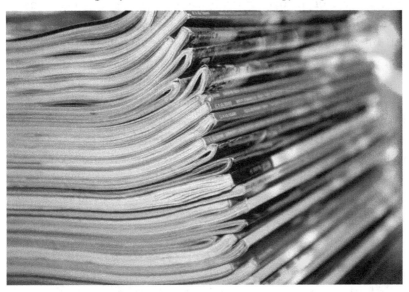

VOLATILE SOLVENTS: TOLUENE

More than any other hazardous air pollutant, toluene is emitted into the air in large quantities from industrial sources where solvents for cleaning and degreasing, and automotive fuels are produced. Toluene is ranked 25th on the list of top chemicals produced in the United States. Those with the highest occupational exposure work in the fields of shoemaking, painting, printing, and automotive production. Toluene is naturally present in emissions from forest fires and volcanoes.

INDOOR AIR EXPOSURE

As a vapor in the air, toluene can be emitted from a number of indoor sources, including building and renovation materials, furniture, art supplies, and cigarette smoke. Studies confirm that toluene is common in indoor air across the United States and can also occur from printed matter, as toluene emissions from magazines continue beyond their manufacturing. Magazines that are stored in homes contribute to indoor concentrations, depending on the storage time and conditions, the number of magazines, and the length of reading time and use of the magazines. Because magazines stay closed most of the time they retain toluene vapors. It is assumed that roughly 60% of the toluene is still in the magazine at disposal. Newsstands and pressrooms show high concentrations of toluene, and the use of personal copiers also increases the level of toluene in indoor air.

Absorption takes place via inhalation and is distributed to the liver, lungs, brain, kidneys, adrenal glands, skin, bone marrow, and white adipose tissue, and passes through both the placenta and breast milk. Because elevated toluene vapors are found nearer the ground, children are exposed to higher levels of toluene than adults.

Noted Health Effects

Human studies indicated that acute exposure to toluene is neurotoxic, affects visual and motor skills, cognitive functioning, and is also toxic to the reproductive system. Higher doses and brain concentrations can accurately predict changes in neurophysiological function and in behavior. The combination of alcohol and toluene exposure can affect the liver more than either can alone, and when combined with aspirin, toluene exposure can increase ill effects on hearing.

Potential effects on hormonal imbalances and reproduction are concerning. Limited information has suggested a connection between spontaneous miscarriages in women occupationally exposed to toluene, as well as when fathers had exposure even when mothers did not.

Safety Classification

The United States Environmental Protection Agency categorizes toluene as a Group D carcinogen – inadequate evidence to classify.

VOLATILE SOLVENTS: XYLENE

Xylene refers to a mixture of three compounds: meta (m-), para (p-), and ortho (o-). Most commercial xylene is a mixture of the three, while it may also contain toluene and benzene. Xylene is one of the top 30 chemicals manufactured in the United States, and in 2006 over 18 billion pounds of xylene was produced. It is used in the manufacture of plastics and Mylar, and in the production of the polyester fiber Dacron. It is also an ingredient used in fabric and paper coatings. Xylene is used as a solvent in the leather, rubber and printing industries, and as a cleaning agent or thinner for paints and varnishes. It is also found in small amounts in gasoline and in aviation fuel.

HUMAN EXPOSURE

Symptoms related to xylene exposure include irritation to the eyes, throat and nose, headache, nausea, vomiting, dizziness, weakness, tremors, irritability or giddiness, lack of muscle coordination, confusion, and ringing in the ears. Other documented effects include balance problems, a decrease in numerical ability, impaired reaction time and short-term memory, and possible changes in the kidneys and liver.

SAFETY CLASSIFICATION

In humans, no information is currently available on the carcinogenic effect of xylene. The Environmental Protection Agency has categorized xylene as "not classifiable as to human carcinogenicity."

VOLATILE SOLVENTS: HEXANE

n-Hexane, a chemical solvent and byproduct of gasoline refining, was introduced in the 1930s as an efficient and inexpensive technique to extract proteins from soy. n-Hexane is also used in the textile and printing industries, to manufacture special glues for the roofing and shoe industries, and in the furniture and leather industries. It is used as a solvent for varnishes, inks, and glues, and as a degreasing agent in the printing industry. Several hundred million pounds of n-hexane are produced each year in the United States.

Environmental Exposure

The United States Environmental Protection Agency tightly monitors and controls n-hexane, considering it a hazardous air pollutant, and heavy fines are imposed for its excessive release. However, 19 million pounds of n-hexane were released into the atmosphere in 2009, with more than two-thirds coming from soy processing plants in the manufacture of health products, with petrochemical plants and tire factories making up the rest of the emissions. n-Hexane can create ground-level ozone when reacting with other air pollutants, also posing health hazards.

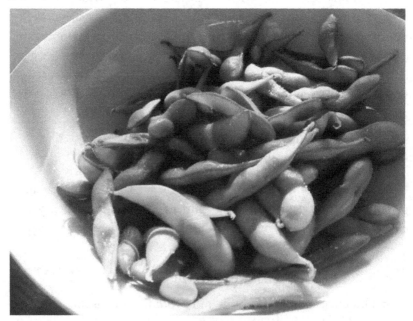

The Soy Industry

Research led by the Cornucopia Institute exposed the soy industry's n-hexane manufacturing process in 2009, and since that time many prominent natural foods companies have changed their extraction method to hydraulic expeller pressing. This process extracts 25-45% less soy protein and isolates than n-hexane does, but companies such as Spectrum Naturals and Turtle Island Foods believe it is more environmentally responsible.

n-Hexane is not an ingredient or raw product; it is considered a processing aid and is therefore not listed on the food label. Consumers must be aware that when contacting companies to inquire about n-hexane processing, they can receive misleading answers. No ingredient can be derived from n-hexane, so careful interpretation should be used if the company states their soy is not n-hexane-derived – the real question is whether or not an n-hexane-extraction process is *used*. Some companies are not even aware their raw materials were exposed to n-hexane when purchasing soy from large suppliers. Careful interpretation must be exercised if the company informs consumers that they don't use n-hexane to process soybeans, because it doesn't occur in their own food processing plants. n-Hexane processing is prohibited in foods labeled organic.

The de-fatting process for soy is typically carried out with n-hexane. In this method, soybeans are bathed in n-hexane to separate the protein from the soybean oil. In the final stages of soy processing, n-hexane is steamed out of the protein, but trace amounts of n-hexane are still present in the food. Extra virgin olive oil has reported residual concentrations as high as 19.1 to 95.3 mg/L.

The FDA does not set a limit for n-hexane residuals in food and does not require testing for residues by manufacturers. However, n-hexane residual levels greater than 10 ppm are prohibited by the European Union. The Cornucopia Institute in the United States found n-hexane residuals in soy foods with levels as high at 21 ppm.

SAFETY CLASSIFICATION

The Centers for Disease Control and Prevention has designated n-hexane as a neurotoxin.

Health effects are more than likely related to recurrent exposure over time, and depend on the size and timing of the dose. Toxicity is generally associated with chronic exposure. The charts below can help determine where exposure to VOCs may occur, and health concerns possibly related to them. The final section provides resources and suggestions to reduce exposure.

OCCUPATIONS WHERE POSSIBLE VOC EXPOSURE MAY OCCUR:

Airfreight and transportation operations

Biomedical laboratory technician, hospital staff

Body shop, auto repair/servicing facility, rust preventatives, auto showroom, or automotive industry

Cement production and asphalt roofing manufacturing

Cleaning agents, dry cleaning

Explosives, fireworks

Factory where construction materials are produced: carpet or fabric/leather treatments, paint, glue, solvent, varnish, thinners, shellac, lacquer, adhesives, resins, lubricants, degreasers, or in wood processing

Firefighters

Food packaging worker

Furniture industry

Hairstylist, nail technician, work in a salon

Involved with transportation and storage of petroleum products

Iron, steel, aluminum casting

Leather tanning, leather or textile industries

Maintenance worker

Manufacture of polyester fibers, Dacron, nylon, or other synthetic fibers

Manufacture of boats, refrigerators, bathtubs, or shower enclosures or open mold processes

Manufacture of car seats, cushions, foam bedding, refrigerators

Manufacture of cleaning supplies and detergents

Manufacture of dyes, perfumes, synthetic fragrances, nail polish

Manufacture of inner tubes and tires, or other rubber industry

Manufacture of polyurethane, plastics, Mylar, foams, fiberglass

Mining, coal manufacturing, coke oven workers

Paper coating, fabric coating

Pesticide production

Pharmaceutical manufacturing

Printers, ink and graphite production, copier repairs

Production of paper, plastics, Styrofoam

Recycling plant worker

Shoemakers, shoe shiners, shoe manufacturing, or footwear assembly

Silk-screen printing, die stamping, film processing

Soy processing industry where hexane is used

Taxidermy

Toll station workers

Wood coating facility

Work in a foundry or near incinerators

Work in confined places: trenches, tunnels, garages, warehouses

Work in dentistry

Work in magazine and news printing and handling industries, photocopy worker

Work in the field of construction: painter, builder, floor finisher, carpet installer, work with insulation

POSSIBLE EXHAUST EXPOSURE:

Air travel

Commute in heavy traffic congestion

Drive an older vehicle

Motor boating

Residing close to an airport, bus station, tunnels, parking lots, highways, or other heavily trafficked areas

Ride snowmobiles, motorcycles

Tailgating while driving

Use gas-powered tools – snow blower, mower, chain saw, leaf blower, etc.

POSSIBLE EXPOSURE TO VOCS AT HOME:

Burn candles in the home

Cigarette smoking occurs in the home

Have an attached garage

Living near any type of incinerator or in close proximity to a petroleum manufacturing facility, gasoline station, or hazardous waste site

Near areas of active forest fires and/or active volcano eruptions

Renovated home with new carpeting or have new furnishings; use of paint and paint remover inside the home

Store gasoline, paint, thinners, or varnish in the home

Use a wood stove to heat the home

Use and store cleaning products in the home

Use charcoal lighter fluid for barbecuing

Use glues, adhesives or art supplies without ventilation

Use mothballs and/or air deodorizers in the home

Use natural gas for cooking

Use pesticides inside the home

"New car smell"

Benzene in foods and personal care products (ie. sodium benzoate, benzoic acid)

Cigarette smoking

Consume food or beverages from containers with #6 recycling code

Consume non-organic hexane-processed soy products and vegetable oils

Dry clean your clothing

Eat or drink out of Styrofoam, especially hot food or beverages

Eat with plastic utensils, plates, and cups

Exercise or ride bicycles along roadways

Personal care products and makeup

Reading magazines, storing large amounts in the home

Refueling your car

Showering in or drinking contaminated well water

Teflon cookware

Use a photocopier or computer printer in the home

Use artificial fragrances in the home or car: sprays, plug-ins, candles

Use nail polish, hair dye, or wear perfume

POSSIBLE HEALTH CONCERNS ASSOCIATED WITH VOC EXPOSURE:

Alterations in brain functioning measured by EEG (electro-encephalography)

Asthma, bronchial irritation, cough, or phlegm

Balance and coordination problems

Blood and bone marrow disorders, anemia

Cancer of the lungs, kidneys, bladder

Changes in vision, loss of color vision, blurred vision

Changes liver functioning

Decreased clotting time

Decreased sperm motility

Dermatitis, eczema

Drowsiness or fatigue, weakness

Eye, nose, or throat irritation

Feeling of being drunk

Headache

Health concerns with peripheral nerves (motor and sensory nerves that connect the spinal cord and brain)

Hearing loss, ringing in the ears

Impaired reaction time

Impaired short-term memory

Increased levels of growth hormone, prolactin, and thyroid releasing hormone (TRH)

Irregular menstrual cycle or ovary shrinkage

Irritability, or giddiness

Leukemia, non-Hodgkin's lymphoma, other blood and bone marrow cancers

Lightheadedness, vertigo

Mental confusion

Miscarriage

Nausea, vomiting, stomach pain

Numbness in the extremities

Poor quality sleep

Rapid heart rate

Tremors, muscular weakness

Tumors of the esophagus and pancreas

WITH THESE ACTION STEPS AND BY USING THE
"RESOURCES AND SUGGESTIONS" THAT FOLLOW

Avoid exhaust and reduce children's exposure to exhaust

Avoid nonorganic hexane-processed soy products

Bike on off-road biking paths

Check for a supplier or manufacturer near your home

Check personal care products for safety

Consider air filtration systems for your car, office, or home

Consider glass and stainless steel for food storage and beverages, and explore safe options for disposable dining ware

Consider less hazardous building and renovation products and check your household products for safety ratings

Consider online magazine and newspaper subscriptions

Consider water purification systems

Detoxify regularly

Don't tailgate or let your car idle in an attached garage

Explore the use of houseplants to clean the air

If you currently store chemicals in an attached garage or in the home, move them to a shed

If you smoke, explore smoking cessation programs

If you use well water, consider regular testing

Make sure employers adhere to OSHA guidelines

Read ingredient labels on food

Refrain from the use of artificial fragrances and consider essential oils

Stay one cars' length behind vehicles in traffic

Ventilate your office when using printers, as well as your home hobby area, or during renovations

When barbecuing use briquettes that don't require lighter fluid, such as natural hardwood charcoal

RESOURCES AND SUGGESTIONS

AIR PURIFICATION

The National Aeronautics and Space Administration's (NASA) Clean Air Study published in 1989 revealed certain plants have the ability to clean the air. Plants shown to remove benzene include gerbera daisies, chrysanthemums, peace lilies, bamboo palm, English ivy, and Mother-in-law's tongue. The study is available at **http://ntrs. nasa.gov/archive/nasa/casi.ntrs.nasa.gov/19930073077.pdf.**

For information on the effectiveness and health benefits of air cleaning devices, visit the Lawrence Berkeley National Laboratory at **https://eta.lbl.gov/search/node/air%20cleaners.**

CIGARETTES

If you smoke, do so only outside your home and motor vehicle. The United States Department of Health and Human Services, in cooperation with the National Institutes of Health and the National Cancer Institute, have several programs to personalize your smoking cessation program. By visiting the main website **https://smokefree. gov/**, you can access the following programs by scrolling to the bottom of the webpage for smokefreeVet, smokefreeWomen, smokefreeTeen, smokefreeEspanol, and smokefree60⁺.

Cookware and Paper Products for the Kitchen

Whenever possible, use stainless steel cookware and utensils and refrain from using Teflon cookware. Store leftovers in glass or stainless steel. Use a stainless steel thermos for your coffee -- most coffee shops offer a discount for using your own travel mug or thermos. When purchasing meats on Styrofoam trays, re-wrap in unbleached parchment paper. Better yet, go to the meat counter and they'll wrap it in paper for you.

Explore other options for disposable cups, plates, and utensils. Eco Products features recyclable dining ware made from sugarcane and bamboo. You can access their website at: **http://www.ecoprod uctsstore.com.**

Alternative compostable and recyclable serving containers are available made with wheat straw fiber from World Centric Organization **http://www.worldcentric.org/.**

Databases for VOCs

Check whether or not there is a chemical supplier or manufacturer near your home by visiting **http://www.thomasnet.com** and entering the VOC chemical name (benzene, ethylbenzene, toluene, xylene, styrene or hexane) into the search area. On the results page, you will have an opportunity to select your state to narrow down the search.

The National Library of Medicine, U.S. Department of Health and Human Services website, available at **https://hpd.nlm.nih.gov/**, lists products containing chemicals in the following categories: arts & crafts, auto products, commercial/institutional products, home office, home maintenance, inside the home, landscape/yard, personal care, pesticides, and pet care. One can do a "Quick Search" for the chemical name. On the Search Results page, select the "Primary Record" which will provide brand names of these household products.

The Healthy Building Network website provides a comprehensive database with more than 1,600 building products and 34,000 chemicals to help users avoid the chemical hazards found in building materials and products. Information on the Pharos database is available at: http://healthybuilding.net/content/pharos-v3.

The Agency for Toxic Substances and Disease Registry website provides Toxicological Profiles with information about contaminants. Use the portal to find out more at: https://www.atsdr.cdc.gov/tox profiles/index.asp.

EXERCISE

Explore the Rails to Trails Conservancy website for bike trails traversing through mostly off-road areas. There are over 30,000 miles of trails across the United States that can be searched for by zip code http://www.railstotrails.org/experience-trails.

EXHAUST

When driving, refrain from tailgating to decrease the amount of exhaust you'll breathe from the vehicle in front of you and stay at least one car's length behind the car at traffic lights or while sitting in traffic. It may be useful to re-circulate the air in your car while driving or you may want to consider using a car air sanitizer, such as the portable AirOasis model available at http://www.airoasis.com/shop/air-oasis-mobile-sanifier. When starting your car, back it out of the garage as quickly as possible and move away from the home to lessen chances of VOCs entering the structure. If you use gas-powered tools such as a snow or leaf blower, wear a respirator mask.

FOOD AND BEVERAGES

Check for benzene in your food and beverages by closely reading the ingredients label by searching for the words benzoic acid, benzoate, carboxybenzene, flowers of benzoin, or sodium benzoate.

In addition, try to avoid foods processed with hexane. Visit the Cornucopia Institute website for a copy of their publication containing information on soy bars and meat alternatives manufactured using hexane solvents. It is available at: http://www.cornucopia.org/hexane-guides/nvo_hexane_report.pdf.

OCCUPATIONAL EXPOSURE

If you work in an industry where VOC exposure is likely, visit the United States Department of Labor's Occupational Safety and Health Administration's website at **https://www.osha.gov/dep/index.html**. Select the "A to Z" index just below the search area and find the chemical name alphabetically to learn more about OSHA enforcement protocols. In addition, please visit the Worker's Rights and Employer Responsibilities regarding ventilation at work at **https://www.osha.gov/SLTC/ventilation/**.

The United States Department of Labor's "Safety and Health Topics" features information on working with styrene at **https://www.osha.gov/SLTC/styrene/**.

Lastly, if working with art supplies please visit the Professional Artist website for information on "Ventilating Your Studio" by Louise Buyo. **http://www.professionalartistmag.com/news/2010/apr/12/ventilating-your-studio/**

PERSONAL CARE PRODUCTS

Check personal care products for benzene content at the Environmental Working Group's website. Their Skin Deep database contains more than 73,000 products and can be accessed at **http://www.ewg.org/skindeep/**. An additional database on healthy cleaning products is also available at **http://www.ewg.org/guides/cleaners**. These databases are also available through your app store as EWG Healthy Living. An additional app for determining the safety of cleaning products is "Think Dirty. Shop Clean."

Consider wearing quality essential oils instead of perfume. Oils can also be diffused into a room. Refrain from burning candles inside the home, as well as the use of room deodorizers. For information on how to determine what is considered a quality essential oil, visit the National Association for Holistic Aromatherapy link at https://www.naha.org/assets/uploads/The_Quality_of_Essential_Oils_Journal.pdf.

WATER PURIFICATION

If you drink water from or bathe in well water, make sure to regularly test the quality of your water. The Centers for Disease Control and Prevention website has links to information on testing at http://www.cdc.gov/healthywater/drinking/private/wells/.

If living in a heavily contaminated area, the use of a home water filtration system is suggested. A list from the Public Health and Safety Organization shows NSF (National Sanitation Foundation) certified drinking water filters certified to reduce a number of contaminants, available at http://info.nsf.org/Certified/DWTU/Listings.asp?TradeName=&Standard=053&ProductType=&PlantState=&PlantCountry=&PlantRegion=&submit3=SEARCH&hdModlStd=ModlStd.

Water purification systems are available that remove most contaminants. For general information on water filtration and distillation systems, visit http://www.reactual.com/home-and-garden/kitchen-products-2/best-countertop-water-filter.html.

The Aqua Pure Filters website notes that activated charcoal filtration and reverse osmosis systems will remove 97 – 99% of pesticides from water. Filter AP-DW70 removes chlorine, pesticides, and VOCs. See other filters and systems at http://www.aquapurefilters.com/contaminants/150/pesticides.html.

Sweetwater Home Water Purification Systems website features systems for well water, kitchen water, reverse osmosis, and a whole house water filtration system at http://cleanairpurewater.com/.

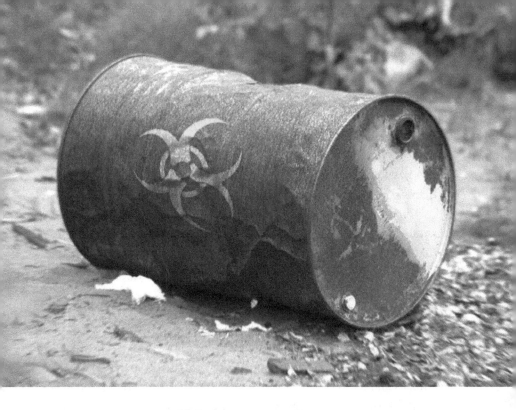

Chapter 2

BANNED BUT PERSISTENT PESTICIDES:

Chlorinated Pesticides

The specific role of a pesticide is to destroy, prevent, or control pests or unwanted species of plants using insecticides (insects), herbicides (vegetation), or rodenticides (small rodents.) Pesticides are used to kill insects that transfer diseases to animals and humans, or insects or animals that damage food during production, processing, transport, and storage. Often useful insects that pollinate plants can die from these chemicals. Chemicals administered to animals to control pests on or in their body are also forms of pesticides. There are currently over 1,600 pesticides available. Reports indicate that the

United States has exported 3.2 billion pounds of pesticides, mostly to developing countries, that are either severely restricted or forbidden in the U.S., including pesticides designated by the World Health Organization to be extremely hazardous and associated with cancer and having endocrine-disrupting effects. Pesticide use in the United States surpassed 1 billion pounds in both 2006 and 2007.

Organochlorine pesticides have been detected in seawater, ice, air, and in mammals in pristine areas of the Arctic and Antarctic, regions that have never used these chemicals. As glaciers melt, they release persistent organic pollutants that have been deposited over the past several decades.

Hormone Disrupting

Pesticides alter normal hormonal balance in both males and females and can lead to infertility. In 1993 the United States Environmental Protection Agency defined endocrine disruptors as chemicals that "interfere with the synthesis, secretion, transport, binding, action, or elimination of natural hormones in the body that are responsible for the maintenance of reproduction and developmental processes." Endocrine disruptors are typically small molecules that mimic natural steroid hormones and include pesticides, PCBs, bisphenol-A, phthalates, dioxins, and other synthetic substances.

Metabolic Syndrome

Recent studies show that persistent organic pollutants and organochlorine pesticides are consistently and strongly associated with obesity-related metabolic syndrome (abnormalities associated with the development of type 2 diabetes and cardiovascular disease), including dyslipidemia and insulin resistance, impaired fasting glucose, and elevated triglycerides. It has been significantly demonstrated that organochlorine pesticides contribute to peripheral arterial disease, arteriosclerosis, and hypertension in workers who are occupationally exposed to pesticides.

Thyroid Hormones

Structurally similar to thyroid hormones, organochlorine pesticides interfere with the hypothalamic-pituitary-thyroid axis, influencing triiodothyronine (T3), thyroxine (T4), and thyroid stimulating hormone (TSH). Pesticides have also been shown to interfere with iodine uptake by the thyroid. Research on prenatal exposure and infants has focused on the association between thyroid hormones and low birth weight, altered psychomotor and cognitive functioning, and growth retardation. Adequate maternal thyroid hormones are critical to neurodevelopment in early life, as the human fetus does not begin producing sufficient thyroid hormones until week 18 of gestation. Prenatal exposure to hexachlorobenzene and DDE is associated with rapid growth during the first six months of life and being overweight at 14 months of age, while studies also link PCB exposures to elevated Body Mass Index (BMI) in childhood and puberty.

Autism Spectrum Disorders

Endocrine disrupting chemicals are recognized as candidates for risk factors in Autism Spectrum Disorders (ASD) because of their ability to alter hormonal functions that play a strong role in neurodevelopment. Maternal *trans*-nonachlor concentrations were positively associated with autistic behaviors, according to a 2014 study published in *Environmental Health Perspectives*. Maternal urinary concentrations of BPA and phthalates during pregnancy were associated with higher Social Responsiveness Scale (SRS) scores in children ages 7 to 9, scores typical in children with ASD. Other studies report a positive association between maternal DDE levels and SRS scores, and show that PCB exposure in utero is associated with neurobehavioral features of ADHD.

A study conducted in the California's Central Valley showed nearly an 8% increase in ASD symptoms among children whose mothers lived within 1/3 mile of agricultural fields where organochlorine pesticides were applied during days 26 and 81 of their pregnancies. Between 1993 and 1998, researchers examined umbilical cord serum for DDE and PCBs in mothers living near a contaminated Super-fund Site in New Bedford, Massachusetts. The results of the study showed an association between PCBs and pesticides with ADHD-like behaviors.

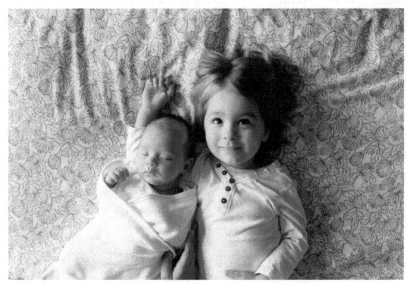

INFANTS AND CHILDREN

For children and infants, diet is a significant source of exposure. Studies have shown that with lower levels of detoxifying enzymes, fetuses and children can't deactivate organic pollutants as easily as adults can, making them more vulnerable to exposure. In 2003 the United States Food and Drug Administration's residue-monitoring program found measureable levels of pesticides in baby foods including DDT and endosulfan.

Pesticides are stored in fatty tissue, so infants are exposed through breast milk when postpartum weight loss increases the release into the milk. Thus, all children are born with a toxic load. In 2004 the Environmental Working Group implemented a study using random samples of cord blood from newborns in the United States. A total of 287 toxic chemicals were detected including 21 pesticides and 147 different PCBs.

Organic Food and Milk

Along with a higher protein quality, when compared with conventionally grown food, organic foods contain fewer pesticide residues but estimates still show that 23% of organic produce samples contain pesticides due to persistent deposits in the soil. A study was conducted using 10 brands of full fat organic milk and 16 conventional full-fat milk samples. Every analyzed sample showed residues of organochlorine pesticides, with hexachlorobenzene showing the most frequent residues. On average, nine pesticides were detected in non-organic milk, and seven in the organic brands. While values of all pesticides were lower in organic milk, DDT was measured in 80% of all samples indicating that contamination by pesticides could not be avoided in organic foods. Endosulfan was present in 50% of the conventional samples, and in 10% of the organic milk.

Cattle are exposed to pesticides through water, feed, and contaminated grasses or pasture, and they make their way into both milk and meat. Cow's milk can also contain higher levels of pesticides following cattle dipping (chemical immersion to control mites, flies, ticks, lice and other parasites.)

In 1996 an herbicide was responsible for killing close to 100,000 fish in Bear Creek, a tributary in Oregon's Rogue River. Analyzing eight urban streams in the United States, researchers detected 116 different pesticides. Bioaccumulation occurs when big fish eat little fish, and humans eat big fish. The concentration of the chemicals in the body increases going up the food chain.

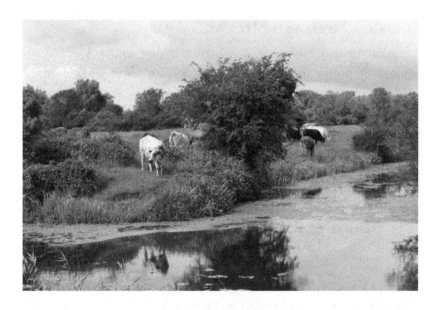

ENVIRONMENTAL AND OCCUPATIONAL EXPOSURE

Human exposure to pesticides also occurs by living close to agricultural areas, or areas that have been treated for health purposes. Golf course fairways and putting greens were found to have 11 different pesticides, and runoff during rainfall resulted in their transport to groundwater. Occupational exposure can occur when employed in the formulation or production of pesticides, or applying them in greenhouses or on agricultural fields, including re-entry, or for pest extermination. Separate studies involving livestock farm workers in Iowa and Ohio reported that flu-like symptoms and respiratory symptoms were significantly associated with pesticide use.

Between 2002 and 2005 in Japan, blood samples from pregnant women were analyzed for 29 pesticides in The Hokkaido Study on Environment and Children's Health. Interestingly 21 of the 29 pesticides detected have never been used in Japan, confirming that highly persistent pollutants can be transported long distances by weather systems resulting in trans-border environmental pollution as they make their way by oceanic and atmospheric currents to their final deposit and accumulation in the Arctic and Antarctic regions. Low temperatures, air jet streams, and sea currents all contribute to high levels of persistent organochlorine pollutants in these isolated zones.

Household Exposure

In the United States 74% of households use an average of between 3 and 4 different pesticides per home, with residues found even on surfaces that have never been treated. Workers in occupations involving the use of pesticides are more likely to carry the chemicals on their clothes, shoes, and skin, and in their vehicles. Chemicals commonly used on lawns also get tracked into the home, and can be detected in bodies of both adults and children. While the half-life of most lawn herbicides is five weeks, they can still be detected in soil one year after treatment. Pesticides are also brought into the home by wind and on pets, and are linked to adverse reproductive effects and cancer in laboratory animals. Inert (forming few or no chemical reactions) ingredients have also been linked to birth defects in humans, liver and kidney damage, and can increase the probability of childhood leukemia and brain cancer.

Noted Health Effects

The association of pesticides with cancer was first noted in the 1960s when farmers using insecticides in grape fields had a higher prevalence of skin and lung cancer. Since then epidemiological and agricultural health studies have associated pesticide exposure to cancer of the brain, breast, colon, esophagus, pancreas, prostate, rectum, stomach, testicles, as well as non-Hodgkin's lymphoma.

These studies also highlight the possible increased risk for leukemia in workers involved in the manufacturing of pesticides. There has also been an increased risk of birth defects observed in children of parents exposed to Agent Orange.

In studies where males were exposed to DDT, decreases in bioavailable testosterone, semen volume and sperm counts were found. Detailed adverse effects of pesticides on the male and female reproductive systems have been noted in a vast body of literature. Among the most reported dysfunctions brought on by pesticides are altered proportion of boys to girls born, changes in pattern of maturity, decreased fertility, demasculinization, elevated rate of miscarriage and testis and ovarian dysfunction.

A growing body of evidence has implicated heritable changes in gene expression with environmental exposures that may be transmitted to future generations and/or serve as a foundation for diseases acquired later in life.

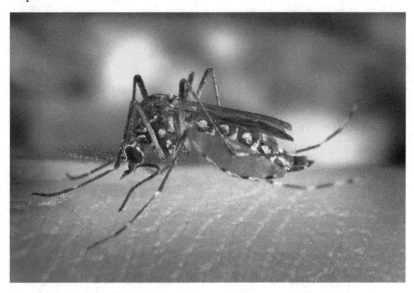

CHLORINATED PESTICIDES: DDT/DDE

DDT was developed by a German chemistry student in 1874, however there was no known use for the compound until 1939 when pharmaceutical researcher Paul Muller of Switzerland was developing an alternative to mothballs and discovered DDT's usefulness as an insecticide. He was awarded the Nobel Prize in medicine in 1948 because of the compound's ability to control disease-bearing insects. During World War II, DDT 's pesticide capability was used to control malaria and typhus. The World Health Organization estimates that 25 million lives were saved with DDT by controlling lice that transmitted typhus and mosquitoes that carried malaria and yellow fever. By 1945 it was put into agricultural use in the United States but, unfortunately, nearly 233 species of insects developed resistance to DDT by 1984. Concerns about bioaccumulation and health effects led to bans throughout the world through the late 1960s to the late 1980s in Australia, Canada, Cuba, Germany, Poland, Sweden, and the United Kingdom. DDT is found around the globe as far as the Arctic and Antarctic, having been carried by atmospheric winds and ocean currents.

Produced in the United States after World War II, DDT was a key ingredient in sprays for lawns and gardens, vegetable dusts, aerosol sprays for flies, a component of kitchen shelf linings to keep food free of beetles, and applied to carpeting to prevent the infestation of fleas. It was also used as a treatment for body and head lice. In 1959 approximately 72 million pounds were produced, peaking at 162 million pounds in 1963. It began to be detected in humans between the 1950s and 1960s. Although prohibited since 1983 China produced approximately 208,000 pounds of DDT between 1991 and 2000, making it one of the largest consumers and producers in the world.

BANNED BUT PERSISTENT

Banned in the United States in 1972, DDT is still found in our environment. An estimated 8,000 – 10,000 pounds of DDT are still being used worldwide to eradicate pests that transmit disease, the most frequent use being in mosquito control.

The biodegradation half-life of DDT in soil is between 2 and 15 years, and up to 20-30 years in some climates. Half-life is the time required for half of the compound to degrade. The amount of residue remaining after a half-life will always depend on how much of the chemical was originally applied. Depending on conditions, DDT applied to soil in 1972 could still have up to 23% of the original amount by 2003.

1 half-life = 50% degraded
2 half-lives = 75% degraded

3 half-lives = 88% degraded
4 half-lives = 94% degraded
5 half-lives = 97% degraded

DDT and DDE (a breakdown product of DDT) remain quite persistent in the environment, especially in cold and temperate climates. They degrade more rapidly in damp, warm conditions and in soil with lesser amounts of sulphate and are considered toxic pollutants due to their increased persistency in the soil and bioaccumulative effect in humans and animals. The consumption of sport fish from the Great Lakes increases DDE and DDT levels in the body, as the half-life of DDT in an aquatic environment is 150 years.

Bioaccumulation in the Body

DDTs are fat-soluble and stored in adipose tissue, the brain, and liver. Estimates show that every 1ppb (parts per billion) of DDT in serum equates to 100-300 ppb in fat cells, 5-10 ppb in the brain, and 47 ppb in the liver. Fatty tissues store DDT and DDE at levels several hundred times that found in blood serum. In addition to breast milk, DDE can be detected in semen, urine, blood, and fat. Long lactation time is associated with lower concentrations of both DDE and DDT in the mother, as they are passed on to the infant via the breast milk.

The half-life of DDT in humans is estimated at 4.2 to 5.6 years and the half-life of DDE is approximately 6 to >10 years, but they tend to continue to increases as a person ages due to cumulative exposure. DDT and DDE are absorbed with dietary fats via the intestinal lymphatic system.

Dietary Exposure

Non-occupational exposure to DDT and DDE occurs by eating contaminated fish, meat, dairy products, dried fruits, and crops grown in contaminated soil, while infants are exposed through breast milk at levels sometimes exceeding what is allowable to be sold commercially in milk products. Milk, cheese and fruit consumers show higher DDE concentrations in the body, while those consuming beef, pork, cold cuts, beer and wine show higher DDT concentrations. Tobacco use has also been related to higher DDE levels.

In addition, people can also come in contact with DDT through residues in airborne dust. Leafy vegetables often contain more DDT because residues in the air are deposited on the leaves. Produce with the highest concentrations of pesticides include apples, broccoli, celery, grapes, green beans, lettuce, peaches, pears, peppers, and strawberries. In the Total Diet Survey, non-organic spinach was the greatest source of DDT in the United States.

According to the United States Food and Drug Administration's Total Diet Study, foods with the highest concentrations of DDE are: farm-raised catfish, non-organic butter, non-organic spinach, Atlantic salmon, American cheese, lamb chops, non-organic collard greens, non-organic cream cheese, and non-organic cheddar cheese. Estimated intakes of DDT/DDE exceeded cancer benchmarks for children, as they consume a greater amount of food and fluids relative to their body weight, and by the age of 12 children were found to exceed a lifetime measure of intake.

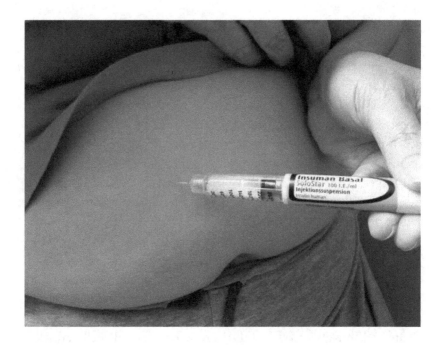

Obesity

All children are exposed in utero and through formula or mother's milk. Recent studies suggested that exposure to DDT in utero can be one of the causes for obesity later in adulthood. Experimental evidence shows certain pollutants promote weight gain and an increase in the development of visceral fat. Data is also linking environmental pollutants with diabetes -- known as diabetogenic pollutants.

Attributing health effects to one specific organochlorine is difficult because exposure to multiple chemicals often occurs. Organochlorine pesticides cross the placenta and act as endocrine disruptors. Adipose tissue in women is remobilized when pregnant in order to supply more nutrients to the developing fetus. The accumulated organochlorides stored in this fat tissue are also mobilized and then pass through the placenta via the blood stream to the fetus. Since older women were children when these substances were banned, these women and those with higher weight gain during pregnancy, or those with no previous pregnancies, have higher DDE concentrations. Tissue specimens collected from 43 placentae at three U.S. locations for a research project conducted by the National Children's Study Placenta Consortium showed every placenta contained DDE, indicating parental exposure.

Hormone Disrupting

DDT is thought to be weakly estrogenic and may bind to estrogen receptors. DDT is believed to act similarly to estradiol. DDE, on the other hand, has potent anti-androgenic activity. Additionally, it has been shown to negatively affect progesterone receptor binding. Studies of menstrual cycles have indicated that DDT and DDE alter menstrual cycles, and increase the risk for early spontaneous abortions. One well-conducted study provided evidence suggesting high DDT exposure is associated with menopause at an earlier age.

Thyroid hormones and DDT/DDE are similarly structured, making it probable that DDT and DDE may interfere with the receptor binding, transport, or synthesis of these hormones. Studies found prenatal exposure to DDT/DDE was associated with increases in thyroid stimulating hormone (TSH) and significant decreases in free thyroxine (fT4), total thyroxine (T4), and total triiodothyronine (T3). Other studies showed associations between higher ratios of DDT/DDE and testicular cancer in male offspring. Testicular cancer is the most diagnosed form of cancer in men between the ages of 20 – 24 years.

Prenatal Exposure and Early Life

Prenatal exposure has been associated with detrimental pregnancy outcomes. Obese mothers typically show higher levels of DDT when compared with underweight mothers due to DDTs affinity for fat. Recent studies indicate that for every natural log unit increase in DDT, birth weight increased by nearly 10 ounces, while DDE exposure decreased both birth weight and gestation time. These chemicals are also thought to exert adverse effects on the mother's thyroid hormone levels, which are essential during the first six months of pregnancy for normal development of the fetal brain. Prenatal exposure can also lead to increased attention problems, a delay in psychomotor and mental development, and decreased cognitive skills evident when children enter preschool.

Growing evidence indicates that when endocrine disrupting chemical (EDC) exposure occurs in early life, an interference with the programming of endocrine-signaling pathways may be altered, including thyroid and steroid hormone functioning. EDCs can also display estrogenic, anti-estrogenic, and anti-androgenic effects. Statistically significant positive associations between prenatal exposure and organochlorides have been associated with higher BMIs at 6.5 years of age. In fact, over 50% of members from both sexes who had ancestral (parent) DDT exposure developed abdominal adiposity and increased body weight even though they had never been directly exposed to DDT. Primary exposure occurred in the U.S. in the 1950s, and three generations have since developed an increasing incidence of obesity.

A study involving 1,455 infants examined whether prenatal exposure to DDE increased wheezing and the risk of lower respiratory infections at 12-14 months old. The results showed that the relationship of DDE concentrations to respiratory issues was statistically significant, increasing risk by 10% as well as increasing risk factors for asthma in children aged 4 and 6 years old.

In a 2007 study, researchers investigated how exposure at different ages can affect disease expression. Studies revealed that women exposed to DDT before the age of 14 showed a 5-fold increase in the risk of breast cancer. In a 2007 study, researchers investigated how exposure at different ages can affect disease expression. They found a significant increase in the risk of breast cancer in the group who were younger than 14 years of age at the time of exposure.

SAFETY CLASSIFICATION

The EPA has classified DDE as Group B2 – a probable human carcinogen.

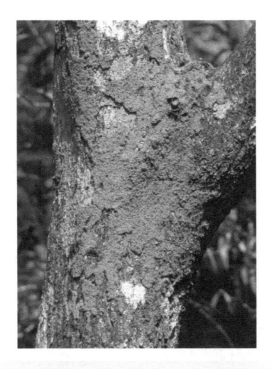

CHLORINATED PESTICIDES:
ALDRIN AND DIELDRIN

From the 1950s until 1970, dieldrin was used as an insecticide on corn, citrus, and cotton, and for timber preservation. It was also used for termite-proofing building boards, plywood, and for rubber and plastic coverings of telecommunication and electrical cables. In 1970, the United States Department of Agriculture terminated all use of aldrin and dieldrin; however, in 1972 the United States Environmental Protection Agency re-approved these insecticides for use in killing termites, thus they remained in use until 1987 when the manufacturer voluntarily canceled the registration. The abbreviated scientific names for aldrin and dieldrin are HHDN and HEOD, respectively.

In plants and animals, aldrin quickly metabolizes to dieldrin. Bacteria and sunlight transform aldrin to dieldrin in the environment. These insecticides bind firmly to soil, slowly evaporate into the air and break down very slowly, remaining unchanged for many years. Plants absorb dieldrin from the soil and store it in their roots and leaves. Although the United States Food and Drug Administration limits residues in raw foods, high concentrations of dieldrin have been detected in squash, butter, heavy cream, cow's milk, carp, trout, and perch.

DIETARY EXPOSURE

Dieldrin is found everywhere in our environment. Exposure occurs by eating fish from contaminated water or by consuming contaminated root vegetables, meat, or dairy products. Root crops such as carrots, turnips, and radishes, are more likely to take up aldrin and dieldrin residues from contaminated soil. According to the FDA's Total Diet Study of Market Basket between 2004 and 2005, foods with the highest concentration of dieldrin are: summer and winter squashes, dill and sweet pickles, cucumbers, pumpkin, farmed Atlantic salmon, cream cheese, peanut butter, and cheddar cheese. Even organic vegetables grown in soil contaminated decades earlier will contain high levels of dieldrin.

PRENATAL EXPOSURE AND EARLY LIFE

These insecticides are found in breast milk and can cross the placenta. High levels of dieldrin were detected in the breast milk of women whose homes were frequently treated with pesticides. Also noted was that dieldrin levels in breast milk continued to rise until the eighth month after treatment of the home was completed. Placental transfer can result in fetal concentrations higher than in maternal blood, increasing the baby's risk from exposure due to immature liver detoxification functioning. Several studies indicate a GABA receptor malfunction and behavioral impairment from in utero exposure in children.

NOTED HEALTH EFFECTS

Health effects can occur after longer periods of exposure to even small amounts, because dieldrin bioaccumulates in the body. Concentrations of persistent organic pollutants increase with age because rates of intake surpass metabolism and excretion. Depending on the amount of the chemical and length of exposure, along with the effects of other chemical exposures, moderate contact of lower doses for longer periods can result in dizziness, headaches, vomiting, nausea, irritability, or uncontrollable muscle movements. Some people can develop a condition where these chemicals cause the body to destroy blood cells. Other adverse health effects include increased rates of Parkinson's disease, hypothyroidism, oxidative damage, and disruption of dopamine transport in the brain. It has also been shown to reduce the production of testosterone, contributing to infertility.

Safety Classification

A common contaminant at hazardous waste sites, the EPA's National Priorities List identifies dieldrin in at least 287 of the 1,613 sites being monitored. Dieldrin occurrence in soil continues to be above state mandated clean up levels in New Jersey, Connecticut, New York, Texas, and California. Based on its current standing with the EPA's Integrated Risk Information System last updated in 1993, dieldrin is classified as Category B2, a "probable human carcinogen." However, the cancer potency for dieldrin is five times that of benzene, with a strong suggestion in studies that dieldrin can cause an increase in risk for developing breast and lung cancer, and non-Hodgkin's lymphoma.

CHLORINATED PESTICIDES: HEPTACHLOR

In 1952 heptachlor was registered in the United State for use on agricultural crops as an insecticide and as a seed treatment. It was also used in homes and on gardens for insect control, including termites. Heptachlor persists in the soils for several years. About 20% of heptachlor is converted into its more harmful metabolite (substance), heptachlor epoxide, both in the body and in the environment within just a few hours. In 1974 all registered uses of heptachlor, expect for termite control and dipping of non-food plants, were cancelled and by March of 1978 most uses of heptachlor ceased. Since 1987 in the United States, heptachlor is still being used to control fire ants. It is applied by adding the chemical into a concrete or metal enclosure and then buried in pad-mounted electric power transformers and in underground telephone and television cable boxes. Velsicol Chemical Corporation in Memphis, TN manufactured and processed heptachlor in the United States. In 2013, the plant, dubbed "The epicenter for wide-ranging environmental problems," was demolished.

Heptachlor is on the United States Environmental Protection Agency's National Priorities List, targeted for long-term federal clean-up activities. It has been detected in at least 129 Superfund Sites, and heptachlor epoxide at 87 sites. Heptachlor is designed to act as a neurotoxicant in insects. In humans and animals, the central nervous system is one of the target systems this compound affects. The liver is also a target organ.

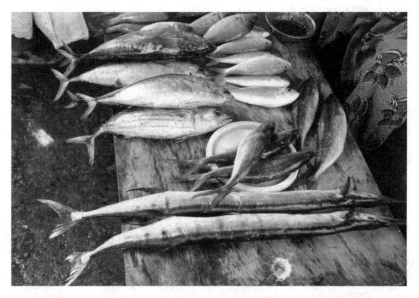

Dietary Exposure

Heptachlor and heptachlor epoxide bind to soil, are immobile and persistent, and bioaccumulate in the food chain. Heptachlor in the air can be deposited on the leaves of plants or can enter the plant from contaminated soil. Animals eat the plants where heptachlor is absorbed and it builds up in their fatty tissue. The half-life of heptachlor in soil is approximately two years, while heptachlor epoxide is very resistant to further chemical changes in the soil. Heptachlors bioaccumulate in fish and animals and is highly toxic to both warm water and cold water fish, as well as waterfowl, game birds, and mammals.

These chemicals have also been detected in dairy products, meat, and poultry, including well water used for drinking in several states. Toddlers and children who drink large amounts of milk may have greater exposure. The FDA's Total Diet Survey detected high levels of heptachlor epoxide in 50% of non-organic butter. It was also detected in 34% of farmed Atlantic salmon and cream cheese, 32% of ground beef samples, 30% of Swiss and cheddar cheese, and 25% of Hubbard squash.

Stored in fat, these chemicals readily cross the placenta and are also transferred through lactation. Studies show that heptachlor epoxide is still measurable in fatty tissue three years after exposure. Ninety-seven percent of adipose tissue samples obtained during autopsies in North Texas showed tissue levels of heptachlor epoxide had not significantly decreased between 1970 and 1988.

Noted Health Effects

Researchers found significant associations with lower infant birth weights in exposed children, along with jaundice, increased learning disabilities, and decreased performance on neurobehavioral tests. In addition, females at puberty had a longer luteal phase and a lower drop in the ratio of estradiol to progesterone after ovulation. The luteal phase (beginning after ovulation and ending when the period begins) is critical for the survival of an early pregnancy. In males, undescended testicles and higher follicle stimulating and luteinizing hormone concentrations were evident

Heptachlor has been shown to bind to cellular estrogen and androgen receptors, and in animal studies heptachlor suppressed estradiol and progesterone concentrations in the blood.

Several reports describe a link between leukemia and adrenal tumors and heptachlor exposure in humans. Suspected adverse health effects in humans are an increased risk of breast cancer, non-Hodgkin lymphoma and Parkinson's disease, an increased rate of atherosclerosis, and cryptorchidism (undescended testicles.) Children with immature and developing organs and the elderly with declining organ functioning will be most vulnerable to toxic substances.

Safety Classification

The International Agency for Research on Cancer has concluded that while evidence for carcinogenicity is sufficient in animals, it is inadequate in humans and is thus classified as a Group 2B chemical.

Heptachlor and heptachlor epoxide have been shown to affect DNA synthesis in human cells in genetic mutation studies. They have been shown to cause cancer and birth defects in laboratory animals. They are classified by the United States EPA as a Class B2, a "probable human carcinogen."

Standard classifications are:
Group A - Human Carcinogen
Group B1 - Probable Human Carcinogen (with limited evidence and inconclusive)
Group B2 - Probable Human Carcinogen (inadequate evidence but far from conclusive)
Group C - Possible Human Carcinogen
Group D - Not Classifiable as to Human Carcinogenicity
Group E - Evidence of Non-Carcinogenicity for Humans

Also, toxicity category 1 indicates the highest degree of toxicity, while category 4 is the lowest.

CHLORINATED PESTICIDES: HEXACHLOROBENZENE

Hexachlorobenzene (HCB) is a fungicide used from the late 1940s until 1984 as a seed treatment for onions, wheat, sorghum, and other grains. It is also considered a pesticide. HCB was used in the manufacture of military materials, aluminum, rubber and dyes. It is currently formed as a byproduct during the production of solvents and pesticides. Until 1977 it was produced at the Hummel Chemical Company in South Plainfield, New Jersey and at the Dover Chemical Company in Dover, Ohio. HCB is found in at least 113 of the EPAs 1,699 sites registered on the National Priorities List. It breaks down slowly in air and is transported long-range distances in the atmosphere.

Although banned for use as a fungicide HCB is still used as an industrial chemical and is a by-product in the production of solvents and wood preservatives. Exposure to HCB rapidly spreads through the blood to fat and other tissues where it remains for years and bio-accumulates.

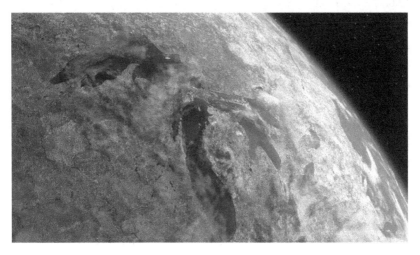

CONTAMINATED WATERS

Hexachlorobenzene adheres to sediment and soil particles, with an initial half-life estimated between three and six years. Research also shows HCB can build up in the bottom of large water bodies such as the Great Lakes. Detailed studies show that the concentration of HCB in Lake Ontario sediment is nearly one million times greater than in its water. Over one half of the HCB added to Lake Erie each year is a result of wet or dry atmospheric deposits. Hexachloroben-zene is listed on the EPA's Great Waters Program as a pollutant of concern due to its ability to persist in the environment, its ability to bioaccumulate, and its toxicity.

Prenatal and Early Life

Hexachlorobenzene transfers from the blood of pregnant women through the placenta to the developing baby, and also transfers through breast milk. Because of its tendency to store in fat, HCB levels in breast-fed babies may be higher than levels in their mothers. HCB also accumulates in people as they age because they are con-tinually exposed to the chemical and excretion from the body is slow.

Dietary Exposure

Most non-occupational exposure to hexachlorobenzene occurs through diet. The World Health Organization's Global Environmental Monitoring Systems/Food Contamination Monitoring and Assess-ment Programme advocates the use of Total Diet Studies (TDS), also known as market basket studies, as a cost-effective method for mon-itoring safe levels of chemicals in dietary intake. Fatty foods typically have higher levels of hexachlorobenzene. The highest levels of HCB were detected in meat, followed by dairy products, fats and oils, and fish. The major food groups contributing to dietary exposure were fish, meats, and cereals. In the United States, 66% of non-organic but-ter samples tested positive for HCB, as did 50% of farmed Atlantic salmon steaks, 41% of lamb chops, 25% of ground beef, and 18% of processed American cheese samples.

Noted Health Effects

Human health effects from hexachlorobenzene exposure include impairment of the thyroid, bone, skin, and liver, and damage to the endocrine, immune and nervous systems. Damage to the kidneys and blood cells have also been observed. Additional adverse health effects of hexachlorobenzene include an increased risk of diabetes, childhood obesity, testicular cancer, soft-tissue sarcomas, thyroid cancers, childhood ear infections, Epstein Barr, chronic fatigue syndrome, autoimmune disorders, non-Hodgkin's lymphoma, and the rare hereditary disease porphyria.

Safety Classification

The United States Environmental Protection Agency has classified hexachlorobenzene as a Group B2 contaminant, a "probable human carcinogen." The International Agency for Research on Cancer categorizes HCB as "possibly carcinogenic to humans," while the U. S. Department of Health and Human Service's National Toxicology Program considers it as "reasonably anticipated to be a human carcinogen." The American Conference of Governmental Industrial Hygienists deems HCB as an A3 carcinogen, "confirmed animal carcinogen of unknown relevance to humans."

CHLORINATED PESTICIDES: MIREX

Between 1959 and 1972, mirex was used as a flame retardant additive (known as Dechlorane) in the manufacturing of plastics, paper, rubber, paint, and electrical goods. As an aerial spray it was also used to kill yellow jacket wasps and fire ants in southeastern United States between 1962 and 1976 as a pesticide. Approximated 132 million acres in North Carolina, South Carolina, Georgia, Florida, Alabama, Mississippi, Louisiana, and Texas were treated with approximately

498,000 pounds of mirex. Between 1957 and 1976, 3.3 million pounds of mirex was manufactured at Hooker Chemical Company located on the Niagara River upstream from Lake Ontario where nearly 6,000 pounds of mirex accidentally entered the Lake. Nease Chemical Company in State College, Pennsylvania also manufactured mirex from 1966 to 1974, while Allied Chemical Company in Aberdeen, Mississippi produced mirex bait.

Previously mirex was also used to control mealy bugs on pineapples in Hawaii, leaf cutter ants in South America, termites in South Africa, and harvester ants and yellow jackets in the western United States. Mirex has been detected at seven of the Superfund Sites listed on the National Priorities List. By 1978 all products containing mirex were banned in the United States.

ENVIRONMENTAL AND OCCUPATIONAL EXPOSURE

Mirex adheres strongly to soil, with a half-life between 10 and 12 years. It can bind to soil particles and travel long distances in water where it is broken down into photomirex by the reaction of sunlight, water, and air. Photomirex is even more toxic than mirex. Mirex has been detected in animals, food, water, sediment, soil, and air, and continues to enter surface water through runoff from contaminated soil, manufacturing facilities, or from leakage at hazardous waste disposal sites. Mirex has been detected in groundwater in agricultural areas in South Carolina and New Jersey. It was also detected in drinking water samples in the Great Lakes area of Ontario, Canada and in Chesterfield County, South Carolina. Plants are contaminated by aerial emissions deposited from the volatilization of mirex from the soil's surface. Uptake and accumulation of mirex has been seen in a variety of plant species. Mirex is toxic to fish.

Human exposure also occurs when living in areas with contaminated soil where mirex was manufactured, disposed of, or sprayed for pesticide application. Occupational exposure is limited to where mirex contamination has occurred or for those involved in clean up and remediation of sites contaminated with mirex.

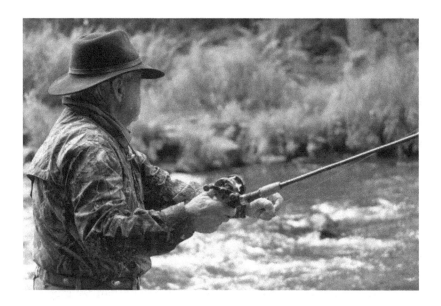

Dietary Exposure

Human exposure to mirex is primarily through food especially meat, wild game, and by eating fish from contaminated water. New York fishermen consuming sports fish from the Great Lakes had serum levels in the 95th percentile for mirex. Currently, Pennsylvania, Ohio, and New York have issued warnings that fish may contain mirex, especially fish from Lake Ontario. Populations living near agricultural communities also show higher concentrations of mirex in blood samples. A study conducted in 2006 showed 86% of pregnant women living near agricultural fields had high levels of mirex.

Noted Health Effects

Mirex is absorbed from the gastrointestinal tract, distributed throughout the body, and stored in fat, leaving the body very slowly. It is also absorbed through the skin. Mirex can cross the placenta and is excreted in breast milk. The main targets of mirex toxicity include the liver, eyes, nervous system, and the developing fetus. Following human exposure, the half-life of mirex concentrations in blood range between three and six months. However, due to its ability to store in fat, mirex will bioaccumulate as the population continues to be exposed at low concentrations.

In humans, mirex causes tiredness, weakness, trembling, and immunological and neurological problems. In laboratory animals, high doses of mirex caused liver tumors and enlargement of the liver, and cancers of the adrenal glands and blood. Testicular damage and decreased fertility were also observed. Edema and cataracts in off-spring was also reported.

SAFETY CLASSIFICATION

The International Agency for Research on Cancer has classified mirex as a Group 2B, "possible human carcinogen." The U.S. Department of Health and Human Service's National Toxicology Program categorizes mirex as "reasonably anticipated to be a human carcinogen."

CHLORINATED PESTICIDES: ENDOSULFAN

Endosulfan is found in at least 176 of 1,699 current or former National Priorities List sites. It was registered for use in 1954 as an effective pesticide against fruit worms, aphids, leafhoppers, beetles, white flies, and moth larvae. Between 1987 and 1997 domestic use of endosulfan was approximately 1.4 million pounds, with 51.4 million pounds used in China between 1994 and 2004.

ENVIRONMENTAL AND OCCUPATIONAL EXPOSURE

Endosulfan travels long distances in the air, as far as the Arctic and Antarctic. Its half-life in soil ranges up to six years. It is considered highly toxic to mammals and birds, showing significant reductions in the number of eggs laid and hatched in birds. The National Oceanic and Atmospheric Agency states that endosulfan killed more fish in the U.S. than all other pesticides between 1980 and 1989.

It is applied as a pesticide to crops grown for food, including numerous types of grains, nuts, fruits, and vegetables. It is also used on cotton plants, tobacco, Christmas tree plantations, and on other ornamental plants. Exposure can occur to field workers as they re-enter orchards or fields that have been treated, or without protective clothing worn while applying the chemical. In addition, they can come in contact with endosulfan by thinning plants, harvesting, pruning, or weeding. Exposure can also occur to workers who handle, mix, load, and apply endosulfan, as well as flaggers who mark the location while the application occurs, or those involved in root dipping. Endosulfan residues have been detected far from application sites in surface waters in California, suggesting exposure to swimmers as well.

DIETARY EXPOSURE

The main source of exposure to endosulfan is from diet. Endosulfan contaminates food and accumulates in the food chain. The food crops most treated are eggplant, squash, sweet potato, cantaloupe, broccoli, pumpkins, pears, tomatoes, potatoes, beans, and peas. In 2007, endosulfan was found in 32 of 40 food samples.

NOTED HEALTH EFFECTS:

Studies indicate a possible association between maternal exposure to endosulfan with thyroid problems and autism in children. Direct exposure of children to endosulfan is related to delayed sexual maturation in males. Exposure also affects the nervous system. The most exposed population is children ages one through six. Endosulfan is transferred to babies through breast milk. It exhibits significant estrogenic activity and can bind to and compete with human estrogen and androgen receptor sites.

SAFETY CLASSIFICATION

The Environmental Protection Agency began taking action to ban endosulfan in the United States in June of 2010 due to its significant risks to agricultural workers and wildlife, and its persistency in the environment. A campaign by the Pesticide Action Network of North

America is promoting a worldwide ban on endosulfan due to concerns that it is a male reproductive toxicant, a carcinogen, and there is abundant evidence of neurotoxicity.

The European Union and the U.S. Environmental Protection Agency both classify endosulfan as Category 1B, highly hazardous. The World Health Organization classifies endosulfan as a priority pollutant.

Health effects are more than likely related to recurrent exposure over time, and depend on the size and timing of the dose. Toxicity is generally associated with chronic exposure. The charts below can help determine where exposure to chlorinated pesticides may occur, and health concerns possibly related to exposure. The final section provides resources and suggestions to reduce exposure.

OCCUPATIONS WHERE POSSIBLE CHLORINATED PESTICIDE EXPOSURE MAY OCCUR:

Employed where solvents, pesticides, and wood preservatives are used or manufactured

Farmers, lawn care and agricultural workers – handling, mixing, loading, and application

Involved with clean up and remediation of sites contaminated with pesticides

Previously worked at Hooker Chemical Company, Nease Chemical Company, Allied Chemical Company, or Velsicol Chemical Company

Work in crawl spaces, basements and ducts in homes treated for termites

Work on electric power transformers, or with underground telephone and television cable boxes where fire ants are problematic

POSSIBLE PERSONAL EXPOSURE TO CHLORINATED PESTICIDES:

Children eating contaminated dirt

Consuming non-organic spinach or dairy products

Consumption of fish from contaminated water

Contaminated ground water, drinking water

Digging around or gardening in soil around foundations previously sprayed for termites

Dwell in a home once treated for termites

High-fat animal food consumption

Live near a hazardous waste site, or in areas heavily sprayed for wasps and fire ants

Not removing clothing or showering before entering the home after occupational exposure

Swimming in contaminated water

Tobacco use

Wearing outdoor shoes inside the home

POSSIBLE HEALTH CONCERNS ASSOCIATED WITH CHLORINATED PESTICIDE EXPOSURE:

Atherosclerosis

Attention problems and decreased cognitive ability in preschool children; behavioral impairment in children

Autism

Blood cell damage

Bone marrow malignancies in children

Breast and testicular cancer

Cerebrovascular disease

Childhood obesity

Delayed sexual maturation in male offspring

Delays in psychomotor development in children

Dizziness, vomiting, nausea, headache

Early menopause

Endocrine gland damage, thyroid problems

Endometriosis, uterine diseases

Epstein Barr, chronic fatigue syndrome

Fatigue, tiredness

Grand-mal seizures

Hormonal imbalances – estrogen, progesterone, testosterone, or thyroid hormones

Immune weakness

Impairment of bone and skin development

Increased risk of cancers: testicular, prostate, breast, thyroid cancers, non-Hodgkin's lymphoma, leukemia, and sarcomas (soft-tissue tumors)

Infertility

Irritability

Kidney damage

Later onset of testicular growth and pubic hair development

Liver abnormalities

Low infant birth weight, jaundice

Lower respiratory infections and asthma in children

Obesity

Parkinson's disease

Poor semen quality

Porphyria (abnormal blood pigment causing dark urine, mental disturbances, and extreme sensitivity of skin to light)

Recurring childhood ear infections

Spontaneous abortions

Type 2 diabetes

Uncontrolled muscle movements

Undescended testicles

WITH THESE ACTION STEPS AND BY USING THE
"RESOURCES AND SUGGESTIONS" THAT FOLLOW

Before purchasing a home, investigate whether pesticides were applied for termite protection, as well as other pesticides that have been used inside the home

Check for a Superfund Site near your home

Check pesticides for safety on the Pesticide Action Network of North America (PANNA)database and the EPA ToxCast website

Check whether there is a mirex manufacturer or supplier near your home

Cook fish and adhere to fish advisories

Detoxify regularly

If pesticides are necessary, consider environmentally responsible products, as well as safer gardening gloves

If you smoke, consider a smoking cessation program

Maintain dust and dirt control in the home, and consider water purification systems

Make sure employers adhere to EPA guidelines and remove shoes and clothing outside of home and shower after working with pesticides

Opt for an organic Christmas tree

Pursue soil testing prior to gardening if living in contaminated areas

Review the Collaborative on Health and the Environment website

Visit The Cornucopia Institute's Egg Score Card

Wash fruits and vegetables before consuming

RESOURCES AND SUGGESTIONS

ALTERNATIVES TO CHEMICAL PESTICIDES

If you must use pesticides in the home or garden, choose traps and baits in place of sprays, or learn more about integrative pest management methods. The Garden's Alive website features environmentally responsible products for insect and pest control, weed control and other categories. It is available at http://www.gardensalive.com under the tab "Natural Pest Control."

CHRISTMAS TREE ALTERNATIVES

For Christmas trees that pose the least risk to your family's health, visit the Beyond Pesticides website for information on where organic tree farms are located http://www.beyondpesticides.org/programs/center-for-community-pesticide-and-alternatives-information/pesticide-free-holidays/christmas.

Cigarettes

If you smoke, do so only outside your home and motor vehicle. The United States Department of Health and Human Services, in cooperation with the National Institutes of Health and the National Cancer Institute, have several programs to personalize your smoking cessation program. By visiting the main website **https://smokefree. gov,** you can access the following programs by scrolling to the bottom of the webpage for smokefreeVet, smokefreeWomen, smokefreeTeen, smokefreeEspanol, and smokefree60+.

Databases for Pesticide Chemicals

The Pesticide Action Network of North America categorizes 101 pesticides as possible endocrine disruptors. It offers a Pesticide Database that allows users to search by chemical or product name, and is available at **http://www.pesticideinfo.org/.**

A full listing of genotoxic (destroys genetic material) chemicals are detailed on the EPA ToxCast Website, **https://www.epa.gov/ chemical-research/toxicity-forecasting.**

Check whether or not there is a chemical supplier or manufacturer near your home by visiting **http://www.thomasnet.com** and entering the pesticide name into the search area. On the results page, you will have an opportunity to select your state to narrow down the search.

The Collaborative on Health and the Environment website has several links of importance, such as "Environmental Risks" at **https://www.healthandenvironment.org/environmental-health/ environmental-risks/.** The 2011 Toxicant and Disease Database can be accessed at **https://www.healthandenvironment.org/our-work/ toxicant-and-disease-database/,** where one can search for either toxicants or diseases and disease categories associated with chemicals. as well as the link "Health, Diseases & Disabilities."

The Agency for Toxic Substances and Disease Registry website provides Toxicological Profiles with information about contaminants. Use the portal to find out more at: **https://www.atsdr.cdc.gov/tox profiles/index.asp.**

Fish, Egg and Produce Consumption

Organic diets have been shown to significantly lower exposure to pesticides. Washing produce (organic or not) partially removes soil particles and pesticides weakly bound to the surface. The peel is generally more contaminated than the pulp. Trim fatty areas of fish and meat. Cooking beef boiled for 90 minutes reduced DDT by 62%. It has also been shown that raw milk has significantly higher levels of DDT than in UHT (ultra-high temperature processed) and pasteurized milk and that skimmed milk led to slight reduction in DDT.

Reducing exposure to pesticides is possible by decreasing the amount of animal products consumed, substituting organic animal products whenever possible, and selecting the lowest fat option. Trim fatty areas from meat. Cooking beef boiled for 90 minutes reduced DDT by 62%. It has also been shown that raw milk has significantly higher levels of DDT than in UHT (ultra-high temperature processed) and pasteurized milk and that skimmed milk led to slight reduction in DDT.

Pan-frying or deep frying fish with the skin removed can reduce pesticide concentrations by 26 – 35%. Ask at the fish counter if they will remove the skin for you. Advisories for fish consumption are still in effect for the Great Lakes and many other waterways, as the half-life of DDT in an aquatic environment is approximately 150 years. Therefore, adhere to fish advisories and limit fatty fish intake. The National Listing of Fish Advisories is available from the Environmental Protection Agency website at **https://www.epa.gov/fish-tech/national-listing-fish-advisories-general-fact-sheet-2011**, with more information on fish consumption at **https://www.epa.gov/fish-tech**.

The Cornucopia Institute's website hosts an "Organic Eggs Scorecard." It can be found at: **http://www.cornucopia.org/organic-egg-scorecard/**.

Washing produce (organic or not) partially removes soil particles and pesticides weakly bound to the surface. The peel is generally more contaminated than the pulp. Wash hands after handling produce, especially when picking your own in an orchard or field. To clean produce, use cold water from the kitchen faucet and then spray with a diluted vinegar solution and let sit for 5 minutes before rinsing. The recipe Dr. Oz offered for a homemade fruit and vegetable wash was to combine 1 cup water, 1 cup distilled white vinegar, 1 teaspoon of baking soda, and the juice of ½ lemon in a spray pump bottle. There are many different variations of produce washes found on the web, such as http://www.rodalesorganiclife.com/food/veggie-wash.

HOME GARDENING

If you garden wear gloves, but not just any glove. The toxicity of gardening tools is also a problem. The Seventh Generation website hosts information on the topic at http://www.seventhgeneration.com/green-cleaning-household-tips/toxic-gardening-tools-are-growing-problem and provides a link to Healthy Stuff http://www.eco-center.org/healthy-stuff/product-search, a website from the Ann Arbor, Michigan Ecology Center.

For information on soil contaminants and soil testing, visit the University of California Agriculture and Natural Resources page at http://ucanr.edu/sites/UrbanAg/Production/Soils/Soil_Contaminants_and_Soil_Testing/.

Discourage children from playing in or eating soil near foundations, and make sure their hands are washed before eating. When digging in soil around a building where chlordane was applied to protect against termites, use protective clothing as exposure can occur. Remove shoes worn outside before entering home to reduce contamination in the home.

NPL SUPERFUND SITES

The United States Environmental Protection Agency's National Priorities List shows the known releases or threatened releases of hazardous substances, pollutants, or contaminants throughout the United States. Information on current and new proposed Superfund Sites is available at https://www.epa.gov/superfund/national-priorities-list-npl-sites-state.

Occupational Exposure

The US EPA regulates Agricultural Worker Protection Standards regarding pesticides. Visit their website for information on occupational protection, available at: https://www.epa.gov/pesticide-work er-safety/agricultural-worker-protection-standard-wps.

Safety When Using Pesticides

Always follow instructions on the label of any pesticide used in your home or garden. Use a flea comb on pets and launder their bedding often. Spot on treatments (meaning, apply to a "spot" on the pet's skin) for fleas and ticks are safer.

Use chemicals only when necessary and use less toxic pesticides. Read the label carefully and follow directions. If you see "This product is toxic to fish," consider an alternative. Make sure pest application equipment is in optimal working condition, mix correctly, and don't wash spray equipment in rivers, lakes, or ponds. Be aware of any buffer zone when applying near water, and don't apply on windy days. When working with pesticides occupationally, remove shoes and clothing outside of the home, and shower before picking up a child.

If you live in a contaminated area limit contact with soil, plant a dense ground cover or thick lawn, and don't grow produce in the soil.

Water Purification

Avoid bathing in contaminated water. If you drink water from or bathe in well water, make sure to regularly test the quality of your water. The Centers for Disease Control and Prevention website has links to information on testing. It is available at: http://www.cdc. gov/healthywater/drinking/private/wells/.

If living in a heavily contaminated area, the use of a home water filtration system is suggested. A list from the Public Health and Safety Organization shows NSF (National Sanitation Foundation) drinking water filters certified to reduce a number of contaminants, available at http://info.nsf.org/Certified/DWTU/Listings.asp?Tra

deName=&Standard=053&ProductType=&PlantState=&Plant
Country=&PlantRegion=&submit3=SEARCH&hdModlStd=
ModlStd.

Water purification systems are available that remove most contaminants. For general information on water filtration and distillation systems, visit **http://www.reactual.com/home-and-garden/kitchen-products-2/best-countertop-water-filter.html**.

The Aqua Pure Filters website notes that activated charcoal filtration and reverse osmosis systems will remove 97 – 99% of pesticides from water. Filter AP-DW70 removes chlorine, pesticides, and VOCs. See other filters and systems available at **http://www.aquapurefilters.com/contaminants/150/pesticides.html**.

The Sweetwater Home Water Purification Systems website features systems for well water, kitchen water, reverse osmosis, and a whole house water filtration system at **http://cleanairpurewater.com/**.

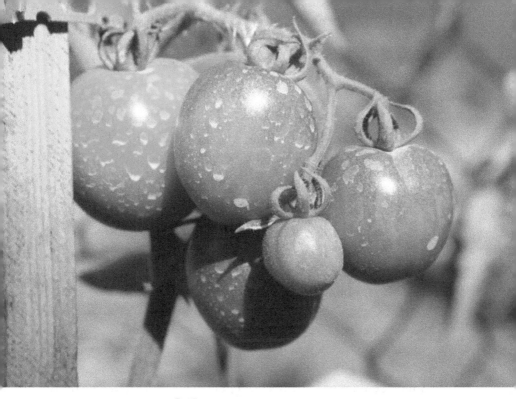

Chapter 3

MOST WIDELY USED PESTICIDES TODAY:

Organophosphate Pesticides

Organophosphate (OP) pesticides are used commercially to control insects on fruit and vegetable crops, as well as on cotton, canola, nuts, and alfalfa. They are also used for home gardening, on certain no-pest strips for flea control on pets, and to treat human head lice. In the past OP pesticides were used inside the home against ants and termites, however these uses are now discontinued. Approximately 32 to 40 OPs are currently used in a variety of formulations in the United States. They are also used in hospitals and schools as a disinfectant, and as a fumigant in sports stadiums, on golf courses or during flower production.

In addition, OPs are used to control yellow fever, malaria, tropical parasites, and diseases. In 2007 approximately 33 million pounds of OPs were used nationwide, accounting for 30% to 36% of all pesticides used in the United States. The use of the OP group of pesticides is cost-effective and they have a wide spectrum of activity.

REGULATING PESTICIDES IN FOODS

Several governmental bodies, including the United States Food and Drug Administration, the United States Department of Agriculture, the United States Environmental Protection Agency (EPA), and the Occupational Safety and Health Organization have developed criteria on levels allowed in foods, the environment, and in the workplace. In 1996 the EPA amended the Food Quality Protection Act to include the Federal Insecticide, Fungicide, and Rodenticide Act, enacted to increase the regulation of pesticide limits in food. Under this act the EPA selected organophosphate pesticides as their first class of chemicals to be reviewed.

The assessment was completed in August of 2006 and resulted in the cancellation of all but a handful of OP pesticides for residential use. A sampling of the EPA's revised guidance shows that the advisory panel allows chlorethoxyfos to be used as a soil application on corn crops; dicrotophos is approved for use on cotton; trichlorfon can be used as a pour-on treatment for beef cattle; and tetrachlorvinphos is to be used only in controlling fecal flies in livestock feed. In addition, the updated summary also listed foods with the highest OP exposure most frequently consumed by children, with snap beans topping the list followed by watermelon, tomatoes, potatoes, pears, and apples.

Lastly, the assessment listed foods treated with the OPs by region:

CENTRAL VALLEY, CA

- Azinphos methyl – almonds, walnuts, apples, pears
- Chlorpyrifos – alfalfa, almonds, walnuts, apples, pears, peaches, apricots, nectarines, asparagus, corn, grapes, sugar beet, tomato

- Dichlorvos – peaches, apricots, nectarines
- Diazinon – almonds, walnuts, apples, pears, peaches, apricots, nectarines, broccoli and other brassicas, cantaloupe, grapes, tomato
- Dimethoate – alfalfa, pears, peaches, apricots, nectarines, broccoli and other brassicas, cantaloupe, corn, legume, tomato
- Disulfoton – asparagus
- Malathion – alfalfa, asparagus, legumes, tomato, corn, grapes
- Methidathion – apples, pears, peaches, apricots, nectarines, almonds, walnuts
- Methyl parathion – alfalfa
- Naled – almonds, walnuts, peaches, apricots, nectarines, grapes, legumes, sugar beet
- Oxydemeton-methyl – broccoli and other brassicas, cantaloupe, sugar beet
- Phorate – corn, sugar beet
- Phosmet – almonds, walnuts, apples, pears, peaches, apricots, nectarines, alfalfa

South FL

- Chlorpyrifos – corn, citrus
- Diazinon – lettuce, tomato
- Phorate – corn, sugarcane

Red River Valley, MN/ND

- Chlorpyrifos – sugar beet, wheat
- Dimethoate – potato
- Phorate – sugar beet
- Terbufos – sugar beet

Mississippi River Valley, MS/LA

- Chlorpyrifos – corn
- Dicrotophos – cotton
- Dimethoate – corn, cotton
- Disulfoton – cotton
- Malathion – cotton
- Methyl parathion – cotton, soybean
- Phorate – cotton
- Terbufos – corn

Eastern NC

- Chlorpyrifos – corn, peanut, tobacco
- Dimethoate – cotton
- Disulfoton – cotton
- Phorate – cotton, peanut
- Terbufos – corn

Willamette Valley, OR

- Azinphos-methyl – apples, cherries, pears
- Chlorpyrifos – apples, cherries, pears, hazelnut, broccoli, cabbage, onions, sweet corn, mint, Christmas trees, nursery, grass for seed
- Diazinon – apples, cherries, pears, snap beans, broccoli, cauliflower, onions, peas, berries
- Dimethoate – cauliflower, peas, cherries, Christmas trees
- Disulfoton – broccoli
- Malathion – apples, cherries, blueberry, onion, squash, raspberry
- Methidathion – pears
- Methyl parathion – onions
- Naled – broccoli, cauliflower
- Oxydemeton-methyl – cabbage, Christmas trees
- Phosmet – apples, cherries, pears

Central Hills, TX

- Chlorpyrifos – alfalfa, corn, cotton, sorghum
- Dimethoate – corn, cotton, wheat
- Malathion – cotton
- Methyl parathion – alfalfa, cotton
- Phorate – cotton
- Terbufos – corn

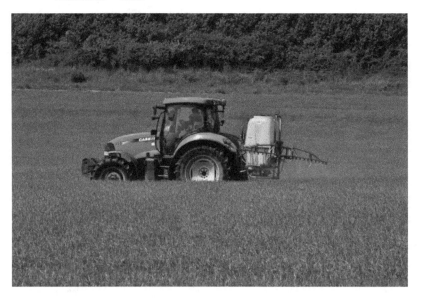

CHLORPYRIFOS

Chlorpyrifos has been detected in at least 7 of the current or former NPL sites. It's unknown how many sites have been evaluated for this and other substances, so as more sites are evaluated the number may increase. In 1997 the manufacturer of chlorpyrifos, Dow Elanco, voluntarily withdrew the chemical for most pet and indoor uses to control termites, fleas, and cockroaches, and also as an active ingredient in tick and flea collars for pets. It is still used in commercial pesticides, such as Lorsban and Dursban, and is used on farms as both a spray on crops and to control ticks on cattle. The EPA recommends a waiting period of 24 hours before re-entering fields where chlorpyrifos was sprayed. Once in the body it passes from the intestines into the bloodstream and is distributed throughout the body. Dermal exposure can occur in infants crawling or laying in an area sprayed with chlorpyrifos.

DIAZINON

Diazinon is found in 25 of the former or current NPL sites. It is used to control insects on fruit and vegetable crops, and on ornamental plants. It is sold only in agriculture under many different trade names, such as AG 500, Alfatox, Basudin, Dazzel, Gardentox, and Knox-out. As of 2004 diazinon is no longer approved in home and garden products. It does not bioaccumulate, and is eliminated from the body within 12 days. However, if an individual is repeatedly exposed, its metabolites can be detected in the urine, indicating chronic low level exposure. Diazinon's primary target in the body is the brain and nervous system. In animal studies, diazinon and its breakdown products are transferred to offspring through both the placenta and in milk.

DICHLORVOS

Dichlorvos has been found at 3 of the current or former NPL sites. Nearly one million pounds of dichlorvos was manufactured in the United States in 1984 for use in food storage areas, barns and greenhouses, and in livestock as a parasite control. Veterinarians also use dichlorvos in pets to control parasites. The EPA estimates that approximately 24,000 U. S. workers are occupationally exposed to dichlorvos. The U.S. Department of Health and Human Services has classified dichlorvos as "reasonably anticipated to be a carcinogen;" the International Agency for Research on Cancer categorizes dichlorvos as "possibly carcinogenic to humans;" while the EPA determined dichlorvos to be a Group B1, "probable human carcinogen."

DISULFOTON

Disulfoton has been identified at 7 of the former or current NPL sites. It is used agriculturally as a pesticide on corn and sorghum, on certain fruit, vegetable and nut crops, as well as on small grains and ornamental potted plants. Disulfoton is also used in smaller amounts to control mosquitos in swamps. It is sold under common trade names, such as Frumin, Disystox, Di-syston, and Solvirex. Depending on climate conditions, disulfoton's half-life in soil can reach up to 290 days. Fish accumulate disulfoton in their bodies, reaching levels sometimes hundreds of times greater than levels detected in the water. In the human body, disulfoton's breakdown products create harmful substances more toxic than disulfoton itself, affecting the brain and nervous system. It is carried by the blood to tissues and organs, and can be completely eliminated in exhaled air, feces, and urine in 10 days or less, if exposure does not continue. When chronically exposed to disulfoton, individuals can become nearsighted.

ETHION

Ethion has been detected in 9 of the current or former NPL sites. Over 868,000 pounds of ethion was used in the United States in 1992 for insect control on citrus trees, nut trees, a variety of vegetables and cotton, and also used on turf grasses and lawns. It is sold under many trade names, such as Nialate, Rodicide, and Bladan. Ethion can enter the environment from landfills, leaks from storage containers, from accidental spills, or during transport. Individuals living near a hazardous waste site could also be exposed. It binds tightly to soil with a half-life anywhere from one month to one year, depending on climatic conditions. Once in the body, ethion is carried to organs by the bloodstream. In the liver ethion is converted to an active form called ethion monoxon, which is much less harmful than ethion. It quickly leaves the body in urine and does not bioaccumulate. Ethion can cause neurological dysfunction with chronic exposure.

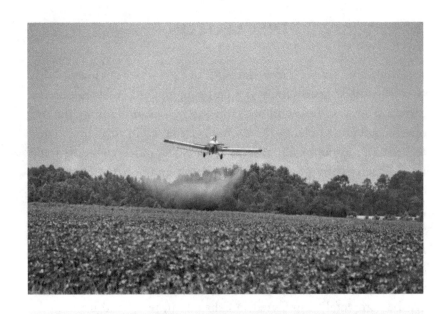

MALATHION

Malathion has been detected in 21 of the former or current NPL sites. It has been manufactured since 1950 in the United States to kill insects on golf courses, in home gardens or on stored food products, where shrubs and trees are grown, and to kill fruit flies and mosquitoes, to treat head lice on humans, and fleas on pets. It is sprayed from airplanes to cover agricultural crops, especially in Florida and California, and has a garlic-like odor. The EPA requires at least 12 hours to pass before a worker's re-entry into fields where the chemical has been applied. If the farmer is hand harvesting or hand pruning, 6 days should pass before re-entry. Malathion remains in the environment for up to several months before being broken down by water, sunlight, and bacteria in soil. It does not break down as quickly on dry soils or man-made surfaces such as pavement, playground equipment, or sidewalks. Those living near farms or NPL sites risk higher exposure, as do individuals living near landfills where malathion has been dumped.

When malathion enters the body it is carried by the bloodstream to organs and tissues, and to the liver for detoxification. Its breakdown metabolites are more harmful than malathion. It does not bioaccumulate and is released through urine. Malathion interferes with normal functioning of the nervous system. The EPA does not have sufficient evidence to classify malathion as a potential carcinogen in humans, although there is evidence suggesting carcinogenic effects in animals. Animal studies have shown that malathion and its metabolites can be transferred through the placenta and milk to animal offspring, but there is no information available in humans.

Concerns exist for exposure to children playing in parks and playgrounds where malathion has been applied. If malathion has been sprayed overhead, there is also concern that children playing in sandboxes will be exposed and caution should be used. It is illegal to use malathion inside the home.

METHYL PARATHION

Methyl parathion has been detected at 21 of current or former NPL sites. Since 1952 it has been manufactured in the United States for use as a pesticide on many kinds of crops and smells like garlic or rotten eggs. It is sprayed on crops from the air, but as of 1999 it is no longer authorized for use on ornamental plants or on crops that children commonly consume including apples, carrots, peaches, pears, and peas. However, it is still used on crops eaten by farm animals and other crops eaten by humans. It is sold under several trade names, such as Vitrex, Thiophos, Soprathion, SNP, Phoskill, Alkron, Folidol, E-605, and Fostox E. Methyl parathion is slow to degrade in the environment, and the EPA recommends a 5-day period before re-entry into fields where it has been applied. Once in the body, methyl parathion travels through the bloodstream to the brain, liver, and other organs. In the liver it is broken down into a more harmful substance called methyl paraoxon. Both methyl parathion and methyl paraoxon can interfere with normal brain and nerve functioning.

ATRAZINE

First registered for use in 1958 in the United States, atrazine is found in at least 20 of the current or former NPL sites. It is sold under several trade names, such as Aatrex, Aatram, Gesaprim, and Atratol but is a Restricted Use Pesticide, meaning only certified users may purchase or apply atrazine. Approximately 76.5 million pounds are applied annually in the United States, with nearly 86% of corn crops receiving treatment. Atrazine kills weeds on highways, near railroads, and on corn, sugar cane, pineapples, wheat, guava, macadamia nuts, sorghum crops, and on evergreen tree farms, golf courses, and near high-voltage power lines.

Contaminated Waterways

After washing from soil into streams it will remain for a very long time and is frequently detected in groundwater and in surface water, especially in the Midwest where it is applied most heavily. It is also used in Florida and the Southeast on residential lawns. Atrazine runoff results in water concentrations that exceed the EPA's concern level as they continue monitoring 17 sites, as of January 2013. The top three priorities are the Youngs Creek and Fabius River in Missouri, and the Big Blue River (Upper Gage) in Nebraska. These sites exceeded what is considered a safe level approximately 5 out of 7 years monitored. In agricultural areas, atrazine is detected in groundwater 40% of the time and 80% of the time in streams. When applied to soil it is washed by rainfall into waterways and can migrate from the soil surface to deeper layers, entering the groundwater and wells. It is suggested that individuals refrain from swimming in lakes, rivers, and streams located near fields where atrazine is being applied.

Atrazine is a persistent organic pollutant, while its metabolite, atrazine mercapturate, is thought to be even more persistent. Atrazine is considered harmful at levels higher than 3 parts per billion, so it doesn't take much to cause problems in the body. An analogy used to describe parts per billion would be to consider that one pinch of salt on 20,000 pounds of potato chips would be the equivalent of 1 ppb. The Nebraskan Big Blue River watershed tested at 148 ppb in May of 2008. Three other watersheds peaked at 100 ppb. Atrazine has been extensively applied in the Great Lakes Basin area. Estimates show that due to run off and atmospheric deposition, the annual input of atrazine to Lake Superior is approximately 2,000 pounds, with 20,000 to 50,000 pounding entering Lakes Erie and Ontario. Atrazine's half-life in the environment is estimated to be 608 days, and 77 years in lakes.

Oftentimes the metabolites of OPs are even more toxic than their parent compounds. For instance, in California's Central Valley malathion and chlorpyrifos metabolites were shown to be 100 times more toxic to frogs than was their primary chemical. Nearly 25% of the OPs used in the United States are concentrated in the Central Valley area, where three and a half million pounds were applied for agricultural purposes in 2008.

Travels Long Distances

Persistent OPs can travel long distances and endure in colder climates, having been detected in both the Arctic and sub-arctic regions. In Svalbard, Norway, five OP compounds were detected in ice core samples. In 2009 the Arctic Monitoring and Assessment Program reported the presence of chlorpyrifos in the Bering & Chukchi seas, in sub-arctic Canadian lakes, in Alaskan fish and snow samples, and in surface water, fog, and ice. Even though OP use has declined, the majority of people in the United States are still routinely exposed.

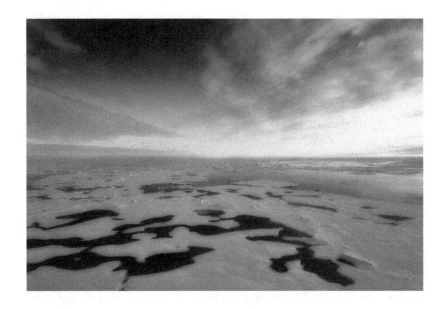

Effects on Insects and Animals

While these chemicals can certainly increase crops by killing bugs, they can also kill beneficial insects, such as bees, as well as animals. The EPA prohibited the use of diazinon in 1988 on sod farms and golf courses due to the destruction of flocks of birds gathering in those areas. OPs have high soil binding, are slightly to moderately soluble in water and most have a low persistence in the environment. Half-lives in non-persistent OPs can range from hours to weeks, while some are known to bioaccumulate in humans and affect the immune, neurological and endocrine systems.

Human Exposure

Human exposure can occur by digging in dirt where atrazine was applied, by drinking contaminated water, ingesting plants containing the compound, or by consuming meat and milk from cattle that have eaten exposed feed or plants. Residues have been detected in wheat, soybeans, sports drinks, and soft drinks. It enters the bloodstream from the lining of the stomach and intestines and is carried to organs and fat.

Nonpersistent OPs can rapidly degrade in air, sunlight and in soil, but chronic exposure still occurs due to the continued use of this class of pesticides on food crops and in food storage centers. Human exposure mainly occurs from ingesting contaminated food and in individuals who work directly with these chemicals. However, exposure can also occur when coming in contact with contaminated dust or air near farms, manufacturing facilities or hazardous waste sites containing OPs, or even the home garden. Powders, shampoos, and sprays used to control fleas and ticks in cats and dogs can contain also OPs.

Individuals may not be aware of previous or ongoing pesticide treatments in their buildings, which include sprays and fogs, and data suggests that exposure may be higher in New York City residents than in the entire United States. Due to the disrepair of buildings in NYC, as well as their density, a reliance on pesticides for indoor use has been deemed necessary. OP pesticides replaced the organochlorine pesticides until 2001 when a shift occurred to using more pyrethroid compounds. Pyrethroids work by disrupting the nervous system of insects, similar to older organochlorine pesticides, and are frequently used on pets and in and around buildings. However, both animal and human studies suggest that pyrethroids may also affect developing nervous systems and reproductive systems.

When applied indoors, OPs are slower to degrade and therefore amplify the risk of exposure. In a 2007 sample of NYC homes, long after OPs were eliminated for indoor use, both chlorpyrifos and diazinon were still detected. DAP metabolites were detected in the urine of over 80% of the 208 residents tested. Time spent indoors in contaminated buildings contributed to exposure concentrations. Seniors typically have 3.8 times more DAP metabolites than adolescents.

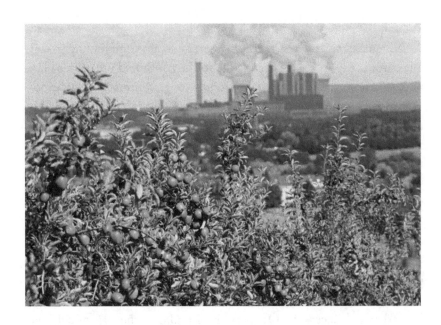

FARM WORKER HOMES

Special attention has been given to farmers and their families. The Child-Specific Aggregate Cumulative Human Exposure and Dose framework was used to study children living in farm worker homes. To estimate exposure levels, children wore socks and union suits that were later analyzed for pesticide loading. In addition to skin contact with OPs, how food was stored and the home's proximity to agricultural fields showed substantial exposure that exceeded the EPA's recommendations in risk assessments.

The Agricultural Health Study reports that members of the farm family can end up receiving a dose of pesticides after the worker applies them. In one case, a farmer applied OP pesticides to pumpkins with a hand-cranked duster. His urinary levels rose three times in magnitude following use, while his spouse and two children showed twice the magnitude of pesticide excretion in their urine. The study also found significantly elevated levels of the organochlorine pesticide dieldrin in six farm families, although the pesticide was banned in the United States in 1987. Other pesticides detected in the families were trans-nonachlor and chlordane, also organochlorine pesticides.

A study conducted on children under six years of age living in the area of a fruit orchard in Washington State showed two highly toxic pesticides not registered for home use. When comparing 46 families living within 200 feet of an orchard, 66% of farm children had DAP metabolite levels four times higher when a family member worked with pesticides, but metabolites were also detected in 40% of nonfarm children living in close proximity to the fields. These children were possibly exposed from food sources, contaminated dust and soil in the area, or through pesticide drift. In 2008 more than 1.6 million pounds of OPs were applied for agricultural purposes in California. In the State's high agricultural areas of Salinas and Oakland, DAP was detected in the dust of 65% - 67% of the homes. Those living in close proximity to sprayed fields showed reductions in whole blood and plasma levels of the neurotransmitter enzyme acetylcholinesterase. Acetylcholine helps to transfer impulses between nerve cells or to other cells, such as in the muscles. If the enzyme (acetylcholinesterase) that breaks it down is inhibited, a buildup of acetylcholine results which leads to overstimulation of the muscles.

Noted Health Effects

Acute exposure levels can result in congestion of the kidneys, lungs and heart, low blood pressure, water retention, adrenal degeneration, and muscle spasms. Chronic exposure above the maximum contaminant level can cause retinal degeneration, cardiovascular damage, reproductive problems, and muscle deterioration. Atrazine increases estrogen production in the body and has been linked to prostate and breast cancers, and non-Hodgkin's lymphoma.

Hormone Disrupting

Some OP pesticides have endocrine disrupting properties, resulting in reproductive disorders, thyroid hormone disruption, an alteration of the pituitary-adrenal and pituitary-thyroid axes, a decrease in testosterone levels, and an increase in prolactin levels. OPs parathion and methyl parathion are estrogen agonists and may interact with receptor sites. Estrogen agonists enhance the activity of estrogen in the body.

An endocrine disruptor, atrazine is known to cause hormonal changes in animals that affect their ovulation and ability to reproduce, including reduced levels of prolactin, luteinizing hormone, progesterone, and testosterone. In his 2010 study, Dr. Tyrone Hayes stated that 10% of male frogs born in water contaminated with atrazine at only 2.5 ppb grew up showing female sex characteristics along with reduced sperm and testosterone levels. The University of South Florida analyzed and published a review of more than 125 studies reporting the same health outcomes, namely that atrazine affected sperm and gonadal development in amphibian species and fresh water fish.

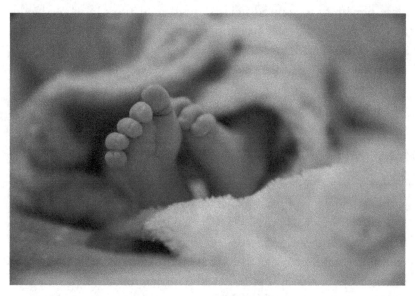

Prenatal and Early Life Exposure

When pregnant women are exposed to atrazine their offspring may develop more slowly and can exhibit birth defects, as well as show damage to the heart, liver, and kidneys. Couples living on farms treated with atrazine had an increase in the risk of pre-term delivery. Data collected between 2004 and 2006 showed shorter gestation in women residing in Kentucky counties with the highest atrazine levels in drinking water. A study conducted in 2009 in Indiana showed that babies with the greatest prenatal exposure to atrazine had lower birth weight. In 1990 Italy banned atrazine due to its presence in water sources. They replaced atrazine with terbuthylazine, which became another chemical concern a few years later. Based on evidence, the European Union banned atrazine in 2001, while in the United States the EPA concluded in 2003, "there is a reasonable certainty that no harm will result to the population" from exposure to atrazine.

Low level, chronic exposure in utero is associated with attention problems, poorer cognitive abilities, and problems with the autonomic nervous system. Children found to have autonomic nervous system dysregulation display more psychosocial and behavioral problems. In the Center for Health Assessment of Mothers and Children of Salinas (CHAMACOS) birth cohort study of 601 women and children, there was a significant association between prenatal DAP exposure and ADHD disorders in children at 5 years of age. In the CHAMACOS study, chlorpyrifos and malathion decreased to undetectable levels when school-age children consumed an organic diet, and returned to higher levels when a non-organic diet was reintroduced. Shorter gestational time and a decrease in fetal growth have also been significantly related to increased urinary OP levels in expectant mothers during late pregnancy. Epidemiological studies report that maternal transfer of OPs to the fetus may occur.

Children can be exposed through soil, pets, dust, and by consuming contaminated foods. They are at higher risk for toxicity than adults because of their limited ability to detoxify harmful chemicals. In addition, the developing brain is more susceptible and the dose per body weight is elevated in children. Fetal exposure to OPs occurs through placental transfer and has been detected in amniotic fluid.

Prenatal and early childhood exposure to OPs has been associated with impairments in short term memory, mental development, working memory, processing speed, perceptual reasoning, verbal comprehension and motor skills, along with abnormal reflexes, increased reaction time, intellectual deficits in middle childhood, and emotional and mental problems developing later in adolescence.

Safety Classification

Most OPs are not classified as carcinogenic, however the Centers for Disease Control do report that several studies are linking exposure to non-Hodgkin's lymphoma and leukemia. OP compounds have also been related to autoimmunity, hypersensitivity, and immunosuppression in those occupationally exposed.

Health effects are more than likely related to recurrent exposure over time, and depend on the size and timing of the dose. Toxicity is generally associated with chronic exposure. The charts below can help determine where exposure to organophosphate pesticides may occur, and health concerns possibly related to OP exposure. The final section provides resources and suggestions to reduce exposure.

OCCUPATIONS WHERE POSSIBLE ORGANOPHOSPHATE PESTICIDE EXPOSURE MAY OCCUR:

Farmers, cattle farmers

Florists, gardeners, greenhouse workers, tree and lawn service

Grounds keeper for golf courses, stadiums, sod farms

Manufacturing of Lorsban, Dursban

Pesticide applicators, those employed in manufacturing of OP pesticides, in their transportation or in mixing or formulating solutions

Previously worked for Dow Elanco

Veterinarian

POSSIBLE ORGANOPHOSPHATE PESTICIDE EXPOSURE AT HOME:

Dwelling in homes treated with OPs

Live near hazardous waste sites, landfills

Live near Youngs Creek or Fabius River in MO; or Big Blue River Gage in NE.

Living near agricultural fields, ie. Willamette Valley, OR; Central Valley, CA; Red River Valley, MN/ND; the Mississippi River Valley, MS/LS; Central Hills, TX; Eastern NC; or Southern FL

Not removing clothing and shoes before entering home after spraying

POSSIBLE PERSONAL EXPOSURE TO ORGANOPHOSPHATE PESTICIDES:

Consuming contaminated produce and fish

Head lice treatment

Pet treatments for ticks and fleas

Playing in sandboxes or play areas treated with malathion

Swimming in contaminated waters, especially in Lake Erie, Ontario, or Superior

POSSIBLE HEALTH CONCERNS ASSOCIATED WITH ORGANOPHOSPHATE PESTICIDE EXPOSURE:

Asthma, wheezing

Attention and behavioral and psychosocial problems in children, learning difficulties, ADHD

Autoimmune disorders

Birth defects – heart, liver, kidneys

Decreased sperm motility and volume, and testosterone, with increased luteinizing hormone

Fatigue, drowsiness

Headache, dizziness, nausea, vomiting, diarrhea

Hormonal imbalance – pituitary, thyroid, adrenal, ovaries, testes

Leukemia, non-Hodgkin's lymphoma, breast or prostate cancer

Low blood pressure, cardiovascular damage

Muscle spasms, deterioration, abnormal reflexes, Parkinson's disease

Nearsightedness, retinal damage

Numbness in the extremities

Poor coordination

Reproductive disorders

Shorter gestation, lower birth weight

Water retention

**WITH THESE ACTION STEPS AND BY USING THE
"RESOURCES AND SUGGESTIONS" THAT FOLLOW:**

Adhere to fish advisories

Check for a Superfund Site near your home

Check for a supplier or manufacturer near your home

Check pesticides for safety on the Pesticide Action Network database and the EPA ToxCast website

Check the Household Product Database for products containing organophosphate pesticides

Consider an organic Christmas tree

Consider soil testing

Consider water purification systems

Detoxify regularly

Do not swim in contaminated water

Dust and sweep often, and consider air purification

Explore options for safer gardening gloves and tools

Grow your own produce

If pesticides are necessary, consider environmentally responsible products

Locate a Farmer's Market near your home or work

Make sure employers adhere to EPA guidelines

Refer to the "What's On My Plate" website for information on the safest produce available in your area

Remove shoes and clothing outside of home and shower after working with pesticides

Visit the Collaborative on Health and the Environment website for more information on pesticides

Wash fruits and vegetables before consuming

RESOURCES AND SUGGESTIONS

AIR PURIFICATION AND DUST CONTROL

The first step is to avoid of exposure and remove known sources from the living environment. Keep dust down in the home if living near areas leading to repeated exposure. Do not wear work shoes inside the home, or any of the clothing worn while applying pesticides, and make sure to shower before entering the home and launder protective clothing outside of the home. Hardwood floors are suggested over carpeting. It may be necessary to sanitize the air and surfaces in your home. Visit AirOasis at **http://www.airoasis.com/** to learn more about NASA developed technology.

For information on the effectiveness and health benefits of air cleaning devices, visit the Lawrence Berkeley National Laboratory at **https://eta.lbl.gov/search/node/air%20cleaners.**

ALTERNATIVES TO CHEMICAL PESTICIDES

If you must use pesticides in the home or garden, choose traps and baits in place of sprays, or learn more about integrative pest management methods. The Garden's Alive website features environmentally responsible products for insect and pest control, weed control and other categories. It is available at http://www.gardensalive.com under the tab "Natural Pest Control."

CHRISTMAS TREE ALTERNATIVES

For Christmas trees that pose the least risk to your family's health, visit the Beyond Pesticides website for information on where organic tree farms are located http://www.beyondpesticides.org/programs/center-for-community-pesticide-and-alternatives-information/pesticide-free-holidays/christmas.

DATABASES FOR PESTICIDES

Check whether or not there is a chemical supplier or manufacturer near your home by visiting http://www.thomasnet.com and entering the pesticide name into the search area. On the results page, you will have an opportunity to select your state to narrow down the search.

The National Library of Medicine, U.S. Department of Health and Human Services website, available at https://hpd.nlm.nih.gov/, lists products containing chemicals in the following categories: arts & crafts, auto products, commercial/institutional products, home office, home maintenance, inside the home, landscape/yard, personal care, pesticides, and pet care. One can do a "Quick Search" for the chemical name. On the Search Results page, select the "Primary Record" which will provide brand names of these household products.

The Pesticide Action Network of North America categorizes 101 pesticides as possible endocrine disruptors. It offers a Pesticide Database that allows users to search by chemical or product name, and is available at http://www.pesticideinfo.org/.

A full listing of genotoxic (destroys genetic material) chemicals are detailed on the EPA ToxCast Website, https://www.epa.gov/chemical-research/toxicity-forecasting.

The Collaborative on Health and the Environment website has several links of importance, such as "Environmental Risks" at https://www.healthandenvironment.org/environmental-health/environmental-risks/. The 2011 Toxicant and Disease Database can be accessed at https://www.healthandenvironment.org/our-work/toxicant-and-disease-database/, where one can search for either toxicants or diseases and disease categories associated with chemicals. as well as the link "Health, Diseases & Disabilities."

The Agency for Toxic Substances and Disease Registry website provides Toxicological Profiles with information about contaminants. Use the portal to find out more at: https://www.atsdr.cdc.gov/tox profiles/index.asp.

Fish Advisories

Advisories for fish consumption are in effect for the Great Lakes and many other waterways. Therefore, adhere to fish advisories and limit fatty fish intake. The National Listing of Fish Advisories is available from the Environmental Protection Agency website at https://www.epa.gov/fish-tech/national-listing-fish-advisories-general-fact-sheet-2011, with more information on fish consumption at https://www.epa.gov/fish-tech.

Visit the website link from the United States Environmental Protection Agency regarding areas of concern in the Great Lakes Contaminated Sediments Program at https://www.epa.gov/greatlakes/contaminated-sediment-great-lakes.

Home Gardening and Soil Testing

The toxicity of gardening tools is also a problem. The Seventh Generation website hosts information on the topic at http://www.seventhgeneration.com/green-cleaning-household-tips/toxic-gardening-tools-are-growing-problem and provides a link to Healthy

Stuff http://www.ecocenter.org/healthy-stuff/product-search, a website from the Ann Arbor, Michigan Ecology Center.

For information on soil contaminants and soil testing, visit the University of California Agriculture and Natural Resources page at http://ucanr.edu/sites/UrbanAg/Production/Soils/Soil_Contami nants_and_Soil_Testing/.

Growing your own produce in a home garden and eating organic as much as possible will reduce your exposure to pesticides. Depending on where you live this might not be possible so on the What's On My Food website (http://whatsonmyfood.org/) one can search by food or by pesticide. For instance, by searching "apples" results indicated 47 pesticide residues were found with data extracted from the USDA Pesticide Data Program. Six of the 47 pesticides were regarded as known or probable carcinogens; 16 suspected of being hormone disruptors; 5 classified as neurotoxins; and 6 categorized as developmental or reproductive toxins, while also indicating that 11 of the 47 pesticides are toxic to honeybees. When searching by pesticide, one is able to find foods currently being treated with the chemical noting the average and maximum levels detected.

LOCAL FARMER'S MARKETS

The United States Department of Agriculture website has a national directory to Farmer's Markets. Searches by state, city, and zip code are available at https://www.ams.usda.gov/local-food-directo ries/farmersmarkets.

NPL SUPERFUND SITES

The United States Environmental Protection Agency's (US EPA) National Priorities List (NPL) is the list of national priorities among the known releases or threatened releases of hazardous substances, pollutants, or contaminants throughout the United States. Information on current and new proposed Superfund Sites is available at https://www.epa.gov/superfund/national-priorities-list-npl-sites-state.

Occupational Exposure

The US EPA regulates Agricultural Worker Protection Standards regarding pesticides. Visit their website for information on occupational protection, available at: https://www.epa.gov/pesticide-worker-safety/agricultural-worker-protection-standard-wps.

Safe Use of Pesticides

Always follow instructions on the label of any pesticide used in your home or garden. Use chemicals only when necessary and use less toxic pesticides. Read the label carefully and follow directions. If you see "This product is toxic to fish," consider an alternative. Make sure pest application equipment is in optimal working condition, mix correctly, and don't wash spray equipment in rivers, lakes, or ponds. Be aware of any buffer zone when applying near water, and don't apply on windy days. If you apply an over-the-counter pesticide yourself, pay careful attention to the instructions on the label. Wear gloves when gardening. You can also be exposed to several OPs by touching grass clippings or other pesticide treated plant materials.

Testing for Pesticide Exposure

Visit Oregon State University's website for information on pest control, pesticide products, and testing for pesticides and pesticide exposure. http://npic.orst.edu/envir/testing.html

Washing Produce

Wash all fruits and vegetables, organic or not, to remove any dirt. Wash hands after handling produce, especially when picking your own in an orchard or field. To clean produce, use cold water from the kitchen faucet and then spray with a diluted vinegar solution and let sit for 5 minutes before rinsing. The recipe Dr. Oz offered for a homemade fruit and vegetable wash was to combine 1 cup water, 1 cup distilled white vinegar, 1 teaspoon of baking soda, and the juice of

½ lemon in a spray pump bottle. There are many different variations of produce washes found on the web, such as http://www.rodalesor ganiclife.com/food/veggie-wash.

WATER PURIFICATION

If you drink water from or bathe in well water, make sure to regularly test the quality of your water. The Centers for Disease Control and Prevention website has links to information on testing. It is available at: http://www.cdc.gov/healthywater/drinking/private/wells/.

If living in a heavily contaminated area, the use of a home water filtration system is suggested. A list from the Public Health and Safety Organization shows NSF (National Sanitation Foundation) certified drinking water filters certified to reduce a number of contaminants, available at http://info.nsf.org/Certified/DWTU/Listings.asp?Tra deName=&Standard=053&ProductType=&PlantState=&Plant Country=&PlantRegion=&submit3=SEARCH&hdModlStd= ModlStd.

Water purification systems are available that remove most contaminants. For general information on water filtration and distillation systems, visit http://www.reactual.com/home-and-garden/kitch en-products-2/best-countertop-water-filter.html.

The Aqua Pure Filters website notes that activated charcoal filtration and reverse osmosis systems will remove 97 – 99% of pesticides from water. Filter AP-DW70 removes chlorine, pesticides, and VOCs, with other filters and systems available at http://www. aquapurefilters.com/contaminants/150/pesticides.html.

The Sweetwater Home Water Purification Systems website features systems for well water, kitchen water, reverse osmosis, and a whole house water filtration system at http://cleanairpurewater.com/.

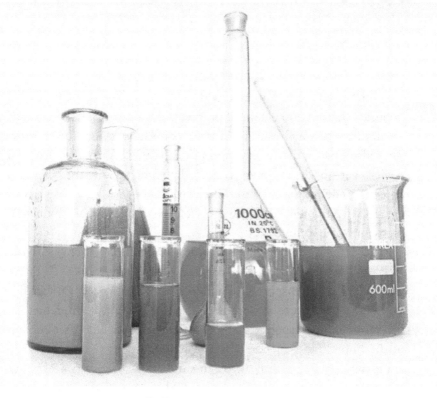

Chapter 4
CHEMICALS USED IN PLASTICS MANUFACTURING:
Polychlorinated Biphenyls (PCBs)

Polychlorinated biphenyls, introduced in the late 1920s, are a class of compounds with chemical and physical properties similar to dioxins. Dioxins, a collective term for a group of environmental contaminants that includes dioxin-like PCBs, are considered a serious and persistent environmental pollutant produced as a byproduct in certain manufacturing processes. There were over 209 PCBs used in manufacturing until it was banned in the mid 1970s, which is when PCBs were first detected in human blood. They are still generated today as byproducts from 200 chemical processes. PCBs are released into the environment through waste incinerators for hospital and solid waste. They also exist in machinery built prior to 1977. When old electrical devices get hot during operation, PCBs enter the air. They can also enter the environment from old electrical transformers, disposal of electrical equipment, and leakage from stockpiles of old industrial lubricants containing PCB.

The United States Environmental Protection Agency's Toxic Release Inventory reported well over 1.6 million pounds of PCBs were released and disposed of in 2007. PCBs are ranked number five on the Priority List of Hazardous Substances for the Comprehensive Environmental Response Compensation and Liability Act section of the Superfund Amendments and Reauthorization Act. There are approximately 275 chemicals on this list, substances of concern that are most commonly found at sites listed on the National Priorities List. PCBs have been detected in at least 500 of the former or current sites on the NPL list.

Between 1929 and 1971 PCBs were manufactured in Anniston, Alabama. Monsanto Company purchased the facility in 1935. The Environmental Protection Agency estimates that 1.4 billion pounds of PCBs were produced before the plant closed in 1971. Court documents show that liquid waste discharged from the plant containing PCBs made its way to Snow Creek at a rate of up to 250 pounds per day, with an additional contribution to air emissions calculated as approximately two pounds per day. In addition, nearly 1 million pounds of PCB-containing waste was deposited into uncapped landfills (finally capped in the 1980s) southwest of the manufacturing facility. Locally raised chickens and hogs showed high levels of PCB contamination, as did fish, leading to a "no consumption" fish advisory set in place in 1990 and that is still in effect today.

FISH AND WATER ADVISORIES

The Environmental Working Group examined farmed salmon that

was purchased in Washington DC, Portland OR, and San Francisco, CA. Farmed fish are closer to shore water, which is the first deposition for run-off from sources of land pollution. They found that PCB levels in all farmed fish samples studied were five times greater than that found in samples of wild salmon. In 1998, 679 fish advisories had been issued in the United States. In 2006, that number increased to 1,023 advisories.

PCB 153's half-life may exceed 100 years on seafloors. Half-life is the time required for half of the compound to degrade. The amount of residue remaining after a half-life will always depend on how much of the chemical was originally involved. The half-lives of PCBs in the human body widely vary by type, ranging from 5 to 15 years or more. PCB 105 has the shortest half-life, while PCB 180 has an elimination rate of 20$^+$ years. The higher the number of the PCB, the more persistent it is in both the environment and in the body.

Canadian advisories are in effect for Great Lakes sport fish due to PCB contamination and recommendations limit fish consumption to 5 ounces per month while pregnant, nursing, or up to five years prior to conceiving. Lake Erie salmon show early sexual development and a loss of secondary male sexual characteristics. Due to PCB contamination, Lake trout became extinct in the 1950s in the Great Lakes and salmon introduced to these waters have shown enlarged thyroid glands.

Of the approximately 2.4 trillion pounds of PCBs produced worldwide, 30% have been discharged into the environment. PCBs persist in the environment for a long time and bioaccumulate in foods, exposing humans to low doses for extended periods of time. PCBs have low solubility in water and deposit in sediment for a remarkably long time. People playing in contaminated water can be exposed when accidentally swallowing water during swimming, or when drinking contaminated well water.

TRAVELS LONG DISTANCES

PCBs are able to travel long distances and have been found in seawater and Arctic snow, far from where they were released. They can travel in the atmosphere as vapor and settle as dust after deposited through snow or rain. Lighter PCBs leave the soil through evaporation and accumulate in the leaves of food crops and plants. Of the 2.4 trillion pounds of PCBs produced worldwide, 400 billion pounds are either waiting for disposal or are still in use. Studies have estimated that the total PCB burden worldwide in soils is 42 million pounds.

Environmental Exposure

The first monitoring site in the United States to test air levels of PCBs was installed in Chicago, IL in 1995. Data showed PCBs have a half-life of three to seven years and are highly influenced by temperatures, with air concentrations measuring 50 to 60 times higher in the summer than in the colder winter months. Both indoor and outdoor levels of PCBs are being monitored in mothers and children in East Chicago, following a dredging project in the Indiana Harbor and Ship Canal that began late in 2012.

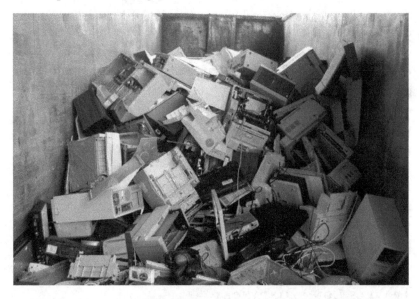

Of the 14 billion pounds of e-waste generated in 1998 in the United States, up to 80% was exported. In 2014 it was reported that most of the world's e-waste (cell phones, computers, appliances, consumer electronics, for example) ends up in China, India, or Africa. An increase in the levels of PCB has been detected in breast milk, blood, and fish in several regions of Africa, attributed to the disassembly and disposal of old transformers, illegal waste incineration, biomass burning, ship dismantling, and increase in e-waste. In 2007, a National Implementation Plan report indicated that some Ghana workers were using empty transformer oil drums as water reservoirs, and that remnant PCB oils were being used to produce a waxy substance used to style hair.

DIETARY EXPOSURE

The most common non-occupational route for human exposure to PCBs is through the consumption of foods from animal origins, accounting for approximately 80%-95% of the body burden. Air emissions result in deposition onto grass, feed, and crops, which are then eaten by animals and humans. In a Belgian study published in 2013, free-range chickens and organic eggs showed higher concentrations of PCBs than from animals raised in battery cages due to the amount of time spent outside and in contact with environment, from consuming contaminated grass, soil, and insects, and the additional exposure to air emissions. Also, free-range animals consume more food on a daily basis to compensate for the additional energy used in running freely outside. Daily foraging can amount to a need for up to 35 grams of food, versus 20 grams of feed for caged animals. The additional exposures result in an increase of dioxins in eggs and meat. The consumption of raw or baked clay around the world and in rural areas of the southeastern United States also increases levels in the body, as clay is highly absorptive of PCBs.

Exposure also occurs through contaminated air or water, and results from natural processes such as forest fires or volcanic eruptions. PCBs are transported long distances and are highly persistent in the environment and in animals and humans. Serum levels of PCBs increase with age due to bioaccumulation, and are higher in those who consume contaminated animal products. Cod liver and fish are found to be the largest contributors of PCBs in the diet, followed by butter, meat, dairy products, eggs, and oils.

Residual amounts of PCBs can be found in feed or applications to the environment surrounding animals. Because PCBs are stored in fat, they are most likely found in food products with high fat content (including breast milk.) The Scientific Committee on Food of the European Union and the Food and Agriculture Organization/World Health Organization Joint Expert Committee on Food Additives and Contaminants has evaluated the toxicity of PCBs and outlined a maximum tolerable monthly intake based on weight. Successive exposure to PCBs results in bioaccumulation, and thus higher levels are detected in those aged 40 and older.

In a study conducted on the PCB content of conventional and organic milk samples in the Canary Islands, PCB-153 and 180 were detected in 100% of the organic milk samples, while PCB-138 was detected in only organic milk. PCB-180 was also measured in conventional milk samples 69% of the time. Interestingly, while organic milks are more highly contaminated with PCBs due to high soil levels swallowed by cows and passed into the bloodstream, conventional milk shows higher levels of organochlorine pesticides. It is important to note, however, that organic standards are formulated by a country's government, so regulations can vary from country to country.

NOTED HEALTH EFFECTS

PCBs are persistent organic pollutants, and although their effects are not completely understood they are linked to health concerns involving the skin and the nervous system. Because PCBs are stored in fat, the lipid-rich brain also attracts these chemicals for storage. PCB compounds were found to be elevated in patients suffering from Parkinson's disease, resulting in a reduction of dopamine and thus affecting motor movement and cognitive functioning. PCBs also interfere with the uptake of the neurotransmitter serotonin.

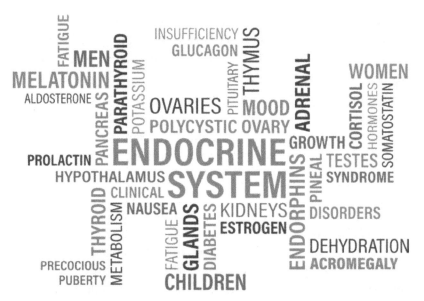

Hormone Disrupting

PCBs are categorized as endocrine disruptors and are associated with decreased thyroid hormone levels, impaired production and development of mature sperm, ovarian dysfunction, endometriosis, abnormal menstrual bleeding, infertility, and alteration of reproductive hormone levels. Concern is growing over low-level prenatal exposure to endocrine disruptors as leading to a decline in fertility in both sexes, an early onset of puberty in females, and delays in male puberty. Between 1960 and 1963 mother's serum samples were collected within 1 to 3 days of a daughter's birth. Researchers recorded time to pregnancy 28-31 years later in 289 daughters. Elevated PCBs in the mother's serum resulted in a 38% drop in the probability of conception and a 30% higher infertility rate in the daughters exposed to PCBs in utero.

Strong evidence suggests that in utero exposure to estrogenic and anti-androgenic endocrine disruptors interfere with reproductive development in male offspring. Some studies show an association of exposure to PCBs with more feminine behavior in boys, and less feminine behavior in girls.

Structurally similar to hormones, endocrine disruptors mimic natural hormones and alter natural functioning. Endocrine disruptors can affect offspring and subsequent generations, possibly leading to transgenerational disease inheritance. A lasting example is prenatal exposure to diethylstilbestrol (DES), a synthetic estrogen used in the 1950s and 1960s to reduce pregnancy complications. Children born to women taking DES have been found to show abnormal gonadal and reproductive tract functioning up to two generations later thus far. Other chemicals thought to affect multiple generations include cocaine, pesticides, and BPA.

THYROID FUNCTIONING

The estrogenic properties of endocrine disruptors can cause an imbalance in estrogen and androgen systems. Non-dioxin-like PCBs can decrease thyroxine concentrations up to 90%, while dioxin-like (although much more potent than non-dioxin-like PCBs) only produce a 40% to 50% decrease in thyroxine levels. Thyroxine is the main hormone made by the thyroid gland. Endocrine disruptors affect genetic programming during early development and have a profound effect on the increased risk of disease in later years, known as the "fetal basis of adult disease." In 2009 the Endocrine Society indicated that endocrine disruptors create a "significant concern for public health."

PRENATAL AND EARLY LIFE EXPOSURE

PCBs are transferred through the placenta to the developing fetus. A critical window of exposure is prenatal life, and PCB-153 was found in 95% of maternal blood samples in several studies. PCBs enter the body and bind to blood lipids. They are then transported via the lipids to the brain, thyroid gland, liver, immune system, and reproductive organs. Increased prenatal concentrations of PCB-153 were significantly associated with lower psychomotor scores in infants, and showed harmful effects on early brain development. Breastfeeding also increases levels during postnatal life as the fat in milk carries these compounds to developing infants resulting in children's blood levels remaining higher during the first months of life.

Attention Deficit Hyperactivity Disorders

It is estimated that 20% of the prevalence of ADHD is associated with exposure to various toxic substances during early development. Researchers found reduced dopamine content in different brain regions, an important factor in ADHD. In addition, researchers have also found that PCBs can inhibit the neural uptake of serotonin, GABA, and glutamate in the brain. Serotonin can affect social behavior, mood, sleep, and appetite. Inuit preschool children with prenatal exposure to PCB-153 exhibited greater states of anxiety and unhappiness.

The maternal body burden can decrease up to 25% during a long period of breastfeeding, but PCBs are then concentrated into the much smaller body of an infant whose diet is exclusively dependent on milk. The effects caused by PCB exposure during the pre- and post-natal period may not appear until many years later.

Immune System Functioning

Little is known about the effects of long-term exposure at low levels and the immune system in humans; however, animal studies show PCB exposure results in immunosuppressive effects and earlier atrophy of the thymus gland. A study conducted on humans in 2014 showed that those with the highest serum level of PCBs had the lowest levels of total white blood cell count, hemoglobin, hematocrit, mean platelet volume, red blood cell counts, lower levels of T lymphocyte counts and INF-gamma levels; while liver enzymes AST, ALT, and GGT were significantly elevated. A study with 207 Dutch children who were three and a half years old, showed prenatal exposure to PCBs was associated with an increased risk of recurrent ear infections, chicken pox and other childhood diseases. New research suggests that PCBs can lower circulating levels of Vitamin D3 in humans.

Obesity

PCBs are also considered potential obesogens, chemicals that act directly on fat cells to increase their number or storage by altering mechanisms that regulate appetite, satiety, and metabolic rate. As endocrine disrupting chemicals, researchers find increasing evidence correlating PCB exposure with leptin resistance and obesity, the incidence of type II diabetes, metabolic syndrome, and cardiovascular disease. PCBs 74, 105, and 118 were all positively related to fat mass in a 2011 study. Women have a higher percentage of body fat than men, and higher body fat percentages are linked to longer half-lives of PCBs.

Safety Classification

PCBs are classified by the International Agency for Research on Cancer as Group 1, a "known human carcinogen." As research continues on the PCB congeners, it is possible they will be re-classified based on toxicological effects, i.e. estrogen receptor antagonists/agonists, immunotoxicant, serotonin inhibitor, or neurotoxicant, for example.

Health effects are more than likely related to recurrent exposure over time, and depend on the size and timing of the dose. Toxicity is generally associated with chronic exposure. The charts below can help determine where exposure to PCBs may occur, and health concerns possibly related to PCB exposure. The final section provides resources and suggestions to reduce exposure.

OCCUPATIONS WHERE POSSIBLE PCB EXPOSURE MAY OCCUR:

Construction (especially demolition of PCB renovation)

Firefighter

Paper manufacturing

Previously employed by Monsanto in Anniston, Alabama

Recycling e-waste

Those working on capacitors and transformers containing PCB

Work in steel production, scrap metal reclamation, smelting, coal combustion

Work with pesticides, herbicides or in their manufacturing

POSSIBLE EXPOSURE TO PCBS AT HOME:

During forest fires or volcanic eruptions

Have well water near Anniston

Live near a hazardous waste site

Live near Snow Creek, or landfills near Anniston, Alabama

Live near the Indiana Harbor Ship Canal, East Chicago

Use fluorescent lighting fixtures, electrical devices, and appliances manufactured prior to 1977

POSSIBLE PERSONAL EXPOSURE TO PCBS:

Consume high fat foods, including butter, dairy, eggs, and meat

Drink contaminated well water

Eating baked clay

Heavy fish consumption

Swim in contaminated water

Work in buildings with PCB sealant materials, caulking

POSSIBLE HEALTH CONCERNS
ASSOCIATED WITH PCB EXPOSURE:

Abnormal behavior, impulsivity, lower IQ scores

Abnormal blood cell counts or liver enzymes

ADD/ADHD, hyperactivity

Advanced pubertal onset in females, delays in male puberty

Anxiety

Childhood asthma, allergies, dermatitis

Children's recurrent ear infections, lower respiratory infections

Decreased attention span, impaired processing speed

Decreased thyroid levels, hypothyroidism

Developmental delay

Diabetes, leptin resistance, obesity

Diabetic nephropathy

Gout

Hyperlipidemia, atherosclerosis, hypertension

Impaired learning and memory, verbal and visual-spatial abilities

Low vitamin D levels

Lymphoma, prostate, testicular, and breast cancer

Non-alcoholic fatty liver disease, liver cancer

Osteoporosis

Parkinson's disease

Polycystic ovarian syndrome, uterine fibroids, endometriosis, abnormal menstrual bleeding, infertility, alterations of hormone levels

Problems associated with motor movement

Reduced semen quality, urogenital tract abnormalities, undescended testicles, higher sex hormone-binding globulin (SHBG) and luteinizing hormone levels, lower testosterone levels in males

WITH THESE ACTION STEPS AND BY USING THE
"RESOURCES AND SUGGESTIONS" THAT FOLLOW

Adhere to fish advisories

Check contamination of fish oil supplements

Check for a Superfund Site near your home

Check for a supplier or manufacturer near your home

Consider water purification systems

Detoxify regularly

Do not swim in contaminated water

If you use well water, consider regular testing

Make sure employers adhere to EPA guidelines

Visit The Cornucopia Institute's Organic Egg Scorecard

RESOURCES AND SUGGESTIONS

DATABASE FOR PCBs

Check whether or not there is a chemical supplier or manufacturer near your home by visiting **http://www.thomasnet.com** and entering "PCB" into the search area. On the results page, you will have an opportunity to select your state to narrow down the search.

The Agency for Toxic Substances and Disease Registry website provides Toxicological Profiles with information about PCBs. Use the portal to find out more at: **https://www.atsdr.cdc.gov/toxprofiles/index.asp.**

Egg Consumption

The Cornucopia Institute's website hosts an "Organic Eggs Scorecard." It can be found at: http://www.cornucopia.org/organ ic-egg-scorecard/

Fish Consumption, and Fish Oil Supplements

The United States Food and Drug Administration sets limits on PCB residues in foods, as does the World Health Organization and European countries. An additional reduction in exposure to PCBs is possible by limiting the amount of animal products consumed, removing the skin of fish prior to cooking, trimming fat from meats, and selecting the lowest fat option in dairy products. If buying fish at a store with a counter, ask them to remove the skin prior to packaging it. Refrain from cooking in lard, butter, or bacon grease, and broil meat and fish so fat drips away.

Adhere to fish advisories. While fish is considered a healthy protein containing essential fatty acids, frequent consumption increases risk, as seafood is a major contributor to dietary intake of PCBs. For fish consumption advisories, visit the Environmental Protection Agency's website at https://www.epa.gov/fish-tech.

Two other useful website links from the United States Environmental Protection Agency regarding PCBs are https://www.epa.gov/pcbs and the Great Lakes Contaminated Sediments Program at https:// www.epa.gov/greatlakes/contaminated-sediment-great-lakes.

PCBs have even been detected in some fish oil supplements manufactured outside of the United States. You may want to search the National Sanitation Foundation Website for safe supplements. It is available at: http://www.nsf.org/services/by-industry/dietary-sup plements/.

NPL Superfund Sites

The United States Environmental Protection Agency's National Priorities List (NPL) shows the known releases or threatened releases of hazardous substances, pollutants, or contaminants throughout the United States. Information on current and new proposed Superfund Sites is available at https://www.epa.gov/superfund/national-prior ities-list-npl-sites-state.

OCCUPATIONAL EXPOSURE

The US EPA regulates Agricultural Worker Protection Standards regarding pesticides. Visit their website for information on occupational protection, available at: https://www.epa.gov/pesticide-work er-safety/agricultural-worker-protection-standard-wps.

WATER PURIFICATION

If you drink water from or bathe in well water, make sure to regularly test the quality of your water. The Centers for Disease Control and Prevention website has links to information on testing. It is available at: http://www.cdc.gov/healthywater/drinking/private/wells/.

If living in a heavily contaminated area, the use of a home water filtration system is suggested. A list from the Public Health and Safety Organization shows NSF (National Sanitation Foundation) drinking water filters certified to reduce a number of contaminants, available at http://info.nsf.org/Certified/DWTU/Listings.asp?Tra deName=&Standard=053&ProductType=&PlantState=&Plant Country=&PlantRegion=&submit3=SEARCH&hdModlStd= ModlStd.

Water purification systems are available that remove most contaminants. For general information on water filtration and distillation systems, visit http://www.reactual.com/home-and-garden/kitch en-products-2/best-countertop-water-filter.html.

The Aqua Pure Filters website notes that activated charcoal filtration and reverse osmosis systems will remove 97 – 99% of pesticides from water. Filter AP-DW70 removes chlorine, pesticides, and VOCs, with other filters and systems available at http://www. aquapurefilters.com/contaminants/150/pesticides.html.

The Sweetwater Home Water Purification Systems website features systems for well water, kitchen water, reverse osmosis, and a whole house water filtration system at **http://cleanairpurewater.com/**.

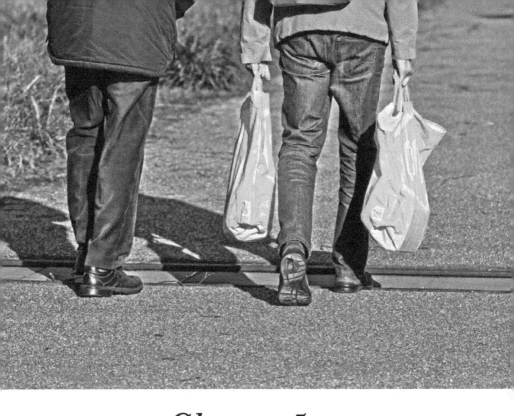

Chapter 5
PLASTICIZERS FOR DURABILITY & TRANSPARENCY:
Phthalates

Phthalates are chemicals that are used to add heat resistance, transparency, durability and plasticity to products manufactured from polyvinyl chloride (PVC.) The annual worldwide production rate of phthalates is several trillion pounds per year. The most widely used phthalate is DEHP [Di-(2-ethylhexly)-phthalate]. Its most notable metabolite is MEHP (Mono-2-ethylhexyl phthalate). MEOHP

[Mono-(2-ethyl-5-oxohexyl) phthalate] and MEHHP [Mono-(2-ethyl-5-hydroxyhexyl) phthalate] are also DEHP metabolites.

Developed in the 1920s, phthalates have been used in the manufacture of a number of consumer goods such as garden hoses, inflatable swimming pools, cosmetics, perfume, toothbrushes, food packaging and films, aspirin, clothing, raincoats, gloves, footwear, artificial leather, pharmaceutical medication and nutritional supplement coatings, toys, lubricants, tablecloths, shower curtains, carpets, vinyl flooring and tile, wallpaper, paint, furniture, insecticides, automobile upholstery, sheathing for wire and cable, laboratory solvents and reagents, blood storage bags, and medical tubing (such as is used in parenteral nutrition and catheters.) Phthalates are easily released from plastic products and thus routes of human exposure include oral, inhalation, ingestion, dermal, and contact with medical devices or vinyl surgical gloves.

ENVIRONMENTAL EXPOSURE

Phthalates are found in the environment and in animals. They are spread in the environment during production, distribution, disposal, incineration of waste containing it, and migrating from consumer products during use. Due to its extensive release into the environment, phthalates have become one of the most abundant industrial pollutants found in sediment, soil, water, and air. Approximately 1.2 million pounds of DEHP was released into the environment from the top 100 US manufacturing companies in 1999. It is estimated that during the same year emissions in Germany exceeded 1.5 million pounds. DEHP has been detected in all fresh water and storm water runoff tested. It has also been detected in ocean sediment and in all the rivers tested in New Jersey. DEHP is one of the most pronounced toxic chemicals in sewage sludge, yet over 5 billion pounds of sludge are spread onto land in the United States annually.

Phthalates have been detected in landfill leachates in Germany, Italy, the United Kingdom, and in the United States. DEHP has been found in Antarctic ice and sub-surface snow at depths of nearly ten feet, as well as detected in jellyfish living in the Atlantic Ocean at depths of 3,000 feet. High concentrations are also found inside buildings with higher temperatures, as the emission of phthalates is associated with increases in temperature.

DIETARY EXPOSURE

According to an assessment by the National Toxicology Program, 90% of DEHP exposure occurs through the consumption of foods that come into direct contact with it either through manufacturing or through migration from food packaging. When volunteers fasted for 48 hours a consistent decrease in urinary metabolites occurred, emphasizing the importance of food exposure to phthalates. Food can become contaminated when exposed to conveyor belts, plastic tubing, coatings on cookware, lid gaskets, plastic gloves worn by workers, and adhesives on food wrappers used in food production, resulting in even organic foods being contaminated with DEHP. Pasta, rice, noodles, and bread have shown to be consistently contaminated with low levels of all phthalates, with canned vegetables and fruits showing significantly higher levels of DEHP than fresh produce.

Foods significantly associated with phthalate metabolite levels include fast foods, poultry, eggs, drinks in plastic bottles, spices, peanut butter, oils, lard, butter, shortening, fish and fish products, and dairy. DEHP contamination was found in lower concentrations in yogurt, and skim and low fat milk, with concentrations up to 100 times greater shown in ice cream, cheese, cream, and whole milk. Because children drink more milk, they are exposed to twice the amount of phthalates than adults. A recent study showed 100% of girls between the ages of 6 and 9 excreted the DEHP metabolites MEHHP and MEOHP, and 94% excreted MEHP, indicating that humans are simultaneously exposed to several phthalates.

A market basket study conducted in New York showed of the 72 commonly consumed foods purchased from Albany, New York grocery stores, phthalates were detected in every sample. DEHP was detected in 74% of the samples, with highest concentrations being found in canola oil, vegetable oil and olive oil packaged in plastic containers.

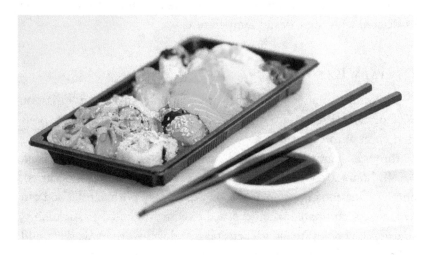

Prenatal and Early Life Exposure

Despite the fact that phthalates do not bioaccumulate, they have been linked to a number of health concerns with exposure beginning in utero and continuing through exposure to breast milk. Phthalate metabolites cross the placenta and have been detected in cord blood, placental tissue, amniotic fluid, and neonatal meconium. Children exposed to phthalates in utero demonstrate more problems with depression and aggression. Prenatal exposure in boys has been associated with reduced masculine play in 3 to 6 year olds.

It is not clear how phthalate metabolites are secreted through the placenta or into different body fluids but it is suggested that they probably have different secretion rates. Phthalates found in the placenta and fetal blood have been shown to have a half-life of 64 hours. Concentrations of certain phthalates detected through biomonitoring studies in the urine of pregnant women has firmly established an adverse association on child behavioral and/or cognitive development, with experimental studies suggesting that prenatal exposure to DEHP alters the transfer of essential fatty acids across the placenta and alters brain development. Phthalates in children's urine shows an association with behavioral problems and reduced IQ. The typical diet of infants has been shown to exceed the Environmental Protection Agency's reference dose - the maximum acceptable oral dose of a toxic substance. Diets high in dairy and meat also exceeded the allowable daily intakes established by the Consumer Product Safety Commission for females.

The function of phthalates is to soften plastic. Soft toys, then, contain higher levels when compared to hard toys. Out of the 24 children's toys studied and purchased from local markets in India, one or more phthalates were detected in every toy. This creates a risk for children mouthing plasticized toys and teethers. Phthalates from the off-gassing of building materials and the migration of PVC flooring to house dust are associated with allergies, asthma, and eczema in children. Urinary levels in early life are also associated with the use of infant formula, breast milk, and cow's milk.

MEDICAL TREATMENTS AND MEDICATIONS

Panel experts from the United States National Toxicology Program, the United States Food and Drug Administration, and Health Canada concluded that while receiving medical care patients are likely exposed to unsafe amounts of DEHP, especially critically-ill infants. Medical care required during a woman's pregnancy can significantly add to her existing levels of DEHP. Of even greater concern is the exposure of infants receiving treatment with DEHP-containing medical devices including ventilator tubes, nasogastric tubes, blood storage bags, parenteral and enteral nutrition tubing and storage bags, and catheters. At this time, the FDA does not require manufacturers to label phthalates on medical products.

Medications are an additional source of exposure to phthalates, with higher levels found in patients taking theophylline (bronchodilator), omeprazole (proton pump inhibitor), didanosine (HIV antiviral), and mesalamine (NSAID). Phthalates are also found in certain laxatives, antihistamines, and antibiotics.

Personal Care Products

In personal care products phthalates help to maintain scents, hold color, dissolve other cosmetic ingredients, and provide flexibility and a moisturizing film – properties that are also useful in the manufacture of fillers, inks, paints, caulks, and adhesives. Phthalates are not bioaccumulative or persistent chemicals, but throughout life humans are continuously exposed through diet, plastic, polyvinyl chloride, and personal care products.

Skin absorption of phthalates from personal care products and cosmetics can be up to 10-times greater on the face than the arm. The Food and Drug Administration found 31 out of 60 personal care products studied contained at least one phthalate. The most common personal care product is deodorant, followed by shampoo and lotion. Researchers found lower levels of urinary phthalates when observing the Old Order Mennonite community located in Germantown, Pennsylvania due to the community's limited use of personal care products. Women who use perfume or cologne show nearly three times higher levels of DEHP, MEHP, and MEHHP. In the United States, there are no regulations in place to mandate the listing of fragrance components and, thus, phthalates are not listed on product labels. Eyeliner, mascara and eye shadow are associated with higher levels of MEOPH. Two brands of denture lining materials exceeded the tolerable daily intake of phthalates for adults by up to 32 times.

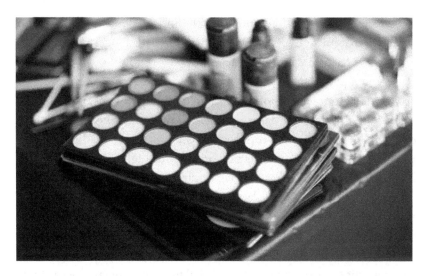

Hormone Disrupting

Acting as a synthetic estrogen, phthalates can influence thyroid hormones, affect bone formation, cause insulin resistance leading to obesity, increase premature breast development and breast cancer, and have been strongly associated with shorter pregnancies resulting in premature births. As previously noted, premature infants are often exposed to plastics during their medical care as well. Studies further support the possibility that prenatal exposure to phthalates may be detrimental to the child's motor and neurodevelopment, and may result in behavioral problems, attention-deficit hyperactivity disorders, reduced scores on IQ tests, social impairment, and somatic complaints including stomach aches and headaches.

Declining fertility is a growing concern. Studies suggest the USA fertility rate fell 45% between 1960 and 2002 with male factors contributing to half of infertility cases. In one study, researchers found that elevated DEHP metabolites showed a negative effect on sperm motility and concentration, and the percentage of abnormal sperm found in men attending a fertility clinic. As researchers report a worldwide decline in the quality of semen, exposure to chemical pollutants has been suggested as a potential risk. Phthalates exhibit anti-androgenic properties resulting in potentially irreversible altered male reproductive development including undescended testicles, smaller scrotum and penis size, and shortened anogenital distance (signifying feminization) in male infants.

In men, phthalate exposure has been linked to distorted levels of free testosterone, estradiol, and follicle stimulating hormone, with reduced sperm motility, damaged sperm, lower sperm counts, prostate damage, and female-like nipples and areolas. Evidence links endometriosis and uterine fibroids in women with high urinary phthalate levels, and shortened gestational duration. Research suggests that maternal exposure to phthalates may affect the sex steroid hormonal status in both the fetal and newborn stages of male and female infants. Premature breast development, sexual development, and earlier first menstruation has been associated with phthalate exposure in young women. Higher urinary levels of phthalates are associated with high blood pressure as shown in a study cohort of 9,756 participants.

A study with 289 individuals conducted by scientists from the Centers for Disease Control found unexpectedly high levels of urinary phthalates in every person tested. Phthalates are eliminated in the urine within 24 to 48 hours, but constant exposure is of concern. One study showed that DEHP was detected in participant's sweat samples but not in serum, suggesting some accrual may be occurring in tissues. A study conducted on normally developing children showed twenty-nine percent of molars tested contained MEHP.

Obesity

Phthalates are associated with an increase in body size. In two cross-sectional studies based on the National Health and Nutrition Examination Survey, a significant association was found between urinary phthalate metabolite concentrations and BMI/waist circumference, including the DEHP metabolites MEHP, MEOHP, and MEHHP. MEHP was associated with increased abdominal fat in children 10 years of age. DiNP, one of the replacement chemicals for DEHP, has been designated by the State of California as a carcinogen. So although DEHP decreased by two to three times over the last twenty years, DiNP exposure appears to have increased four times.

Beginning in 1999 in the United States, every five years six metabolite levels of DEHP are monitored in 5,000 subjects. Large-scale monitoring has also occurred in the German Environmental Survey and through the Canadian Health Measures Survey. NHANES data shows phthalates were detected in 100% of children, and nearly 50% of adults. Included among the top disorders caused by phthalate exposure, data from the Comparative Toxicogenomics Database lists diseases involving the liver and the endocrine, genital, urologic and cardiovascular systems.

SAFETY CLASSIFICATION

The Scientific Committee for Toxicity, Ecotoxicity and the Environment of the European Union classified DEHP as a reproductive and developmental toxicant in 2000. By 2004 the European Union banned six phthalates in children's toys and school supplies. Although phthalates fall under the Toxic Substances Control Act in the United States, they remain basically unregulated in consumer products. However, in September of 2007 the State Senate in California banned 6 phthalates in children's toys, followed by a legislative ban in 2008 by the US federal government. Since 2008, the European Commission has limited phthalates in food contact materials. In 2013, the Office of Environmental Health Hazard Assessment in California added phthalates to the list of chemicals known to cause cancer.

DEHP is included in the International Chemical Secretariat's SIN (Substitute It Now) List due to its classification as toxic to reproductive organs and processes. The World Health Organization's International Agency for Research on Cancer has not yet determined phthalates as carcinogenic to humans. DEHP is classified as an anticipated carcinogen by the National Toxicology Program. The United States Environmental Protection Agency classifies DEHP as B2 – a probable human carcinogen. The Department of Health and Human Services has determined DEHP as reasonably anticipated to be a human carcinogen. Although the FDA does not deem there is enough evidence to regulate phthalates in cosmetics, the Fair Packaging and Labeling Act ensures phthalates must be listed on products, other than fragrances.

Health effects are more than likely related to recurrent exposure over time, and depend on the size and timing of the dose. Toxicity is generally associated with chronic exposure. The charts below can help determine where exposure to phthalates may occur, and health concerns possibly related to phthalates exposure. The final section provides resources and suggestions to reduce exposure.

OCCUPATIONS WHERE POSSIBLE PHTHALATE EXPOSURE MAY OCCUR:

Employed where phthalates or plastics are manufactured or used

Food processing and packaging

Personal care products manufacturing

Polyvinylchloride fabrication workers

Waste management workers, sewage treatment

Wearing surgical gloves

Work in a nail salon

POSSIBLE PERSONAL EXPOSURE TO PHTHALATES:

Baking modeling clay

Children mouthing plastic toys

Consuming certain pharmaceutical drugs and nutritional supplements

Consumption of vegetable oils from plastic containers

Denture lining materials

Diets high in meat and dairy products

Drinking bottled water

Hemodialysis treatments, parenteral and enteral nutrition

Medical devices containing PVC and phthalates

Personal care products, wear perfume or cologne

Plastic food containers, food packaging and films

PVC flooring, shower curtains

Wearing phthalate-containing clothing and footwear

POSSIBLE HEALTH CONCERNS ASSOCIATED WITH PHTHALATE EXPOSURE:

Allergies, asthma, eczema in children

Altered genitals in males, prostate damage, female-like nipples and areolas

Behavioral problems in children, depression, aggression, social impairment

Breast cancer

Elevated blood pressure

Endometriosis, uterine fibroids

Obesity

Premature labor

Premature puberty

Reduced IQ, attention deficit in children

Testicular toxicity, abnormal sperm, reduced sperm motility and quantity

Thyroid hormone imbalance, insulin resistance, elevated sex hormone binding globulin, distorted levels of testosterone, estradiol, follicle-stimulating hormone

EMPOWER YOURSELF

WITH THESE ACTION STEPS AND BY USING THE "RESOURCES AND SUGGESTIONS" THAT FOLLOW:

Avoid containers with #3 recycling code, and bottled water

Check for a supplier or manufacturer near your home

Check personal care products for safety

Consider a water purification system

Consider glass and stainless steel for food storage and beverages, explore safe options for disposable dining ware

Consider less hazardous building and renovation products

Consume low fat animal products

Detoxify regularly

Purchase vegetable oils packaged in glass containers

Refrain from the use of artificial fragrances and consider essential oils

Review the occupational safety guideline for phthalates

Switch to phthalate-free toys

Visit the Collaborative on Health and the Environment website for more information on phthalates

RESOURCES AND SUGGESTIONS

BUILDING AND RENOVATION PRODUCTS

Instead of vinyl shower curtains, purchase those made of polyester or nylon. Avoid plastics marked with #3 recycle symbol, as these plastics are more likely to contain PVC. The Healthy Building Network website provides a comprehensive database with more than 1,600 building products and 34,000 chemicals to help users avoid the chemical hazards found in building materials and products. Information on the Pharos database is available at: **http://healthybuilding. net/content/pharos-v3.**

CHILDREN'S TOYS

For toys that are free of BPA, phthalates, PVC, formaldehyde, and lead visit Mighty Nest at **http://mightynest.com/learn/make-your-nest-mighty/for-your-kids/choosing-safer-toys.** Support toy manufacturers that have pledged to stop using PVC: Brio, Chicco, Early Start, Evenflo, Gerber, Lego, Prime Time, Sassy, and Tiny Love.

DATABASES FOR PHTHALATES

Check whether or not there is a chemical supplier or manufacturer near your home by visiting **http://www.thomasnet.com** and entering "Phthalate" into the search area. On the results page, you will have an opportunity to select your state to narrow down the search.

The Collaborative on Health and the Environment website has several links of importance, such as "Environmental Risks" at **https://www.healthandenvironment.org/environmental-health/environmental-risks/**. The 2011 Toxicant and Disease Database can be accessed at **https://www.healthandenvironment.org/our-work/toxicant-and-disease-database/**, where one can search for either toxicants or diseases and disease categories associated with chemicals. as well as the link "Health, Diseases & Disabilities."

DINING WARE

Do not microwave foods in plastic, and refrain from consuming foods and beverages from plastic cups and dishes. Explore other options for disposable cups, plates, and utensils. Eco Products features recyclable dining ware made from sugarcane and bamboo. You can access their website at: **http://www.ecoproductsstore.com**.

Alternative compostable and recyclable serving containers are available made with wheat straw fiber from World Centric Organization **http://www.worldcentric.org/**.

FRAGRANCE AND ESSENTIAL OILS

Consider wearing quality essential oils instead of perfume. Oils can also be diffused into a room. For information on how to determine what is considered a quality essential oil, visit the National Association for Holistic Aromatherapy link at **https://www.naha.org/assets/uploads/The_Quality_of_Essential_Oils_Journal.pdf**.

Occupational Exposure

If working with phthalates, review occupational safety guidelines at http://www.cdc.gov/niosh/docs/81-123/pdfs/0236.pdf and https://www.osha.gov/SLTC/nailsalons/chemicalhazards.html.

Also review the New Jersey Department of Health and Senior Services handout at http://nj.gov/health/eoh/rtkweb/documents/fs/0765.pdf.

Personal Care Products

Since 2004 over 500 companies voluntarily pledged to remove chemicals of concern from personal care products. To support manufacturers who have signed the "Campaign for Safe Cosmetics" visit: http://www.safecosmetics.org/get-the-facts/safer-cosmetics-companies/campaign-safe-cosmetics-compact-signers/. The Safe Cosmetics Organization has the app, "Think Dirty Shop Clean," which enables one to search over 454,000 products.

The Skin Deep Database from the Environmental Working Group is also searchable online at http://www.ewg.org/skindeep/ or through their app, "Healthy Living." Look for the following ingredients on the label, which indicate the presence of phthalates: DEHP, DEP, DBP, or fragrance, or select products indicating they are "phthalate free." Products labeled "fragrance-free" may still have phthalate-containing agents to mask their chemical odor, whereas products labeled "natural" can also contain phthalates. It's best to check.

Water Purification

Water purification systems are available that remove most contaminants. For general information on water filtration and distillation systems, visit http://www.reactual.com/home-and-garden/kitchen-products-2/best-countertop-water-filter.html.

The Aqua Pure Filters website notes that activated charcoal filtration and reverse osmosis systems will remove 97 – 99% of pesticides from water. Filter AP-DW70 removes chlorine, pesticides, and VOCs, with other filters and systems available at **http://www. aquapurefilters.com/contaminants/150/pesticides.html**.

The Sweetwater Home Water Purification Systems website features systems for well water, kitchen water, reverse osmosis, and a whole house water filtration system at **http://cleanairpurewater.com/**.

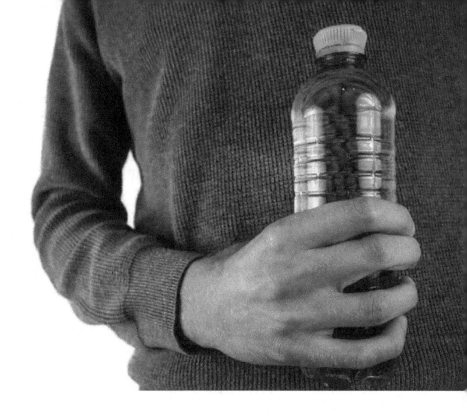

Chapter 6
YET ONE MORE
PLASTICS CHEMICAL:
Bisphenol A (BPA)

First produced in 1891 by Russian chemists, commercial production of bisphenol A (BPA) began in the 1940s and 1950s and it is used in manufacturing polycarbonate plastics for water containers and lids, plastic windows, car bumpers, water supply lines, greenhouses, CDs and DVDs, cell phones, computers, sport and impact-resistant safety equipment, electrical parts, printed circuit boards, and medical devices including IV bags, feeding tubes, and catheters. Its epoxy resins are used to coat cars and boats, water pipes, and food and drink containers. It's also found in many other products including dental sealants, thermal paper receipts, toilet paper, napkins, children's books and toys, pacifiers, baby bottles and nipples, eyeglass lenses and flame retardants.

The worldwide annual production of BPA was estimated to be approximately 10-12 billion pounds in 2011. In 2007, the US EPA's Toxics Release Inventory database showed that the U.S. production volume was estimated at 5.5 million pounds, of which 600,000 pounds were released to air, 30,000 pounds directly to water, 72,800 pounds released on-site to land, and 3.3 million pounds transferred off-site to land. Canada was the first country worldwide to consider BPA a toxic substance. High levels of BPA are found in southern Asia where the burning of plastics for waste disposal occurs. As a result of industrial activity even the Polar Regions show BPA contamination.

Due to the high fat content of brain tissue, the brains of fish along the Allegheny and Monongahela Rivers in the Greater Pittsburgh Area were examined for BPA, resulting in 44 out of 58 samples showing detectable levels. In August of 2012 a study was conducted on both tap water and the main water supply in Madrid. A total of 14 out of 30 endocrine disruptors were found, with flame retardants at the highest concentration followed by BPA. It's important to note that levels were too low to confirm a public health risk but it's also important to remember that these compounds can act at very low doses with effects appearing in the long term.

Human Exposure

Exposure to BPA can occur through consumption of bottled water due to the migration of additives and plasticizers by a diffusion process. A study conducted in 2011 showed that BPA was detected in all bottled water analyzed and although intake fell below legislative values, it contributed to the total daily intake and constant human exposure.

Canada was the first to launch BPA-free baby bottles. However, a report released by Health Canada indicated trace levels of BPA were still detected in bottles marked BPA free. In a study conducted in Europe, 20 out of 27 BPA-free bottles identified release of BPA in migration tests. BPA leaching has been shown to increase when polycarbonate bottles are cleaned with a brush, harsh detergent, or in the dishwasher. The release of BPA from plastic bottles also increases with temperature.

In 2013, Chinese researchers analyzed 287 urine samples of children between 3 and 24 years of age. The detection of BPA in samples was 100%. Participants who used ceramic drinking cups had significantly lower BPA levels than those who used plastic. Urinary BPA levels were significantly decreased when replacing plastic bottled water with boiled tap water and drinking out of ceramic cups. The Centers for Disease Control found detectible levels of BPA in 93% of urine samples from 2,517 subjects over the age of six in the U.S., of which the highest values for daily intake was found in toddlers followed by infants, children, teenagers, and then adults.

DIETARY EXPOSURE

Fatty foods are able to extract BPA from plastics. Four out of five samples studied indicated BPA had leached from plastic containers into olive oil. Because BPA is stored in fat, it has the ability to make its way into breast milk and colostrum. A study conducted on 325 colostrum samples in the U.S. showed nearly 71% had detectable levels of BPA – similar to the BPA detection frequency of 75% in breast milk.

Dietary exposure through food and drink containers is the primary source of human exposure. BPA can leach into food from the coatings of canned foods lined with its epoxy resins especially when heightened by heat, storage time, and storage temperature (such as when kept in a hot garage.) BPA is released from lacquer coatings designed to protect metal cans from corrosion and to protect the food from contamination. However, research shows that exposing tins to temperatures over 212 degrees increases the release of BPA by 18 times. Consuming foods with plastic tableware can also increase the potential of BPA leaching onto foods as can plastic stretch film and reusable plastic food containers.

Exposure through Paper Products

BPA is often used as a developer in paper production so it is also found in paper plates and paper cups, newspapers, magazines, and even toilet paper. A study of 20 brands of kitchen paper towels revealed that those made with virgin paper contained no BPA while paper towels made from recycled paper did, most likely due to the contamination of paper by BPA during the recycling process. Approximately 30% of thermal papers (such as cash register receipts, fax paper, tickets, and ATM receipts) enter paper recycling streams and introduce BPA into the cycle of paper production. It's better to throw these receipts in the trash than it is to recycle them, and also to wash your hands after handling.

In 2008, the National Toxicology Program voiced concern for BPA toxicity in pregnant women and children, while the American Academy of Pediatrics and the Endocrine Society recommends that pregnant women reduce their exposure to BPA and other chemicals. The French Agency for Food, Environment and Occupational Health & Safety committee reported findings that investigations showed a real risk for women who are pregnant, along with risks to their child, when expectant mothers working as cashiers came in contact with thermal receipts that increased BPA levels in their bodies. Data regarding dermal absorption of BPA through the skin shows uptake between 10% and 60%. Thermal receipt papers are produced in large quantities as cash register receipts, luggage tags and airline tickets, for train and bus passes, and lottery tickets. BPA from thermal papers has been shown to be directly absorbed through the skin, and can be ingested after the handling of these papers when transferred by hand to mouth, especially when eating. In 42 supermarket receipt samples collected in China, one receipt sampled contained at least one thousand times more BPA than the amount of BPA found in the epoxy lining of a food can.

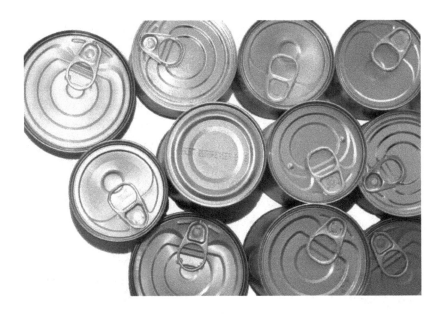

Air and Dust Exposure

Sources of human exposure include both outdoor and indoor air and dust ingestion. BPA was found in 95% of the dust samples analyzed from locations in the Eastern United States and in 86% of house dust samples of 120 Cape Cod homes in Massachusetts. Researchers also collected indoor dust samples from homes in Kentucky and New York between 2006 and 2010. Of the 56 samples analyzed, 95% samples showed elevated levels of BPA. Higher concentrations have been shown in offices due to electronic equipment and printed circuit boards used in electronics.

In a study involving 257 preschool children, researchers found BPA in more than 50% of indoor air, solid food and liquid samples at daycare centers. BPA in floor dust samples showed elevated levels in daycare centers studied in Ohio and North Carolina. Ingestion of dust by toddlers shows the same exposure level used in animal studies that gives rise to health effects.

Prenatal and Early Life Exposure

Levels of BPA have been reported to be elevated in premature infants, and that prenatal and postnatal exposure could impair future adult glucose homeostasis (a balance of glucagon and insulin that maintains blood glucose) by altering the timing or development of the pancreas and the quality and quantity of b-cell populations. B-cells (beta cells) store and release insulin. Premature infants show almost twice the 95th percentile of the general population's BPA levels due to the medical products found in the neonatal intensive care unit: IV bags, tubing, umbilical catheters, and incubators. Those undergoing hemodialysis are also exposed to BPA contained in medical equipment. During dental work BPA can leach into saliva. Depending on the number of crown restorations completed on molars, dental materials may be a relevant source of BPA with the worst case scenario still showing elevated concentrations five days after surgery.

BPA has been detected in urine, blood, amniotic and follicular fluid, placental tissue, breast milk, colostrum, semen, umbilical cord blood, saliva, and adipose tissue. Some studies have suggested that along with an increase in cancer, cardiovascular disease and diabetes, BPA increases externalizing behaviors (lashing out and defiance) in 2-year-olds, especially in female children. Gestational BPA exposure has been shown to be associated with anxiety, hyperactivity, and increased aggression.

NOTED HEALTH EFFECTS

BPA's lipophilic (having a strong affinity for fat) property may result in an accumulation in bodies. There are over 150 published studies on low-dose effects of BPA in animals. These studies indicate BPA toxicity increases certain cancers, genital malformations, earlier vaginal opening, changes in sex characteristics and behaviors, increased aggressiveness, and changes in reproductive and immunologic functioning, among other effects. Along with its ability to affect reproduction and development, both animal and human studies have indicated that BPA can be a causal effect of prostate cancer, cardiovascular disease, neurobehavioral complications, and liver enzyme abnormalities.

Hormone Disrupting

Studies have further shown BPA to be an endocrine disruptor, mimicking estrogenic actions in the body while also having anti-androgenic activity and disrupting the function of leptin, insulin, and thyroxine. Human studies have shown an increase in endometriosis and breast cancer in women, alterations in thyroid and pituitary function, prostate and testicular cancers in men, reduced male fertility, declined semen quality, increased sperm DNA damage, abnormal sexual development, premature puberty, premature labor, reduced birth weight, increased male genital abnormalities, asthma, polycystic ovarian syndrome, recurrent miscarriages, attention deficit hyperactivity, neurobehavioral effects, and immune suppression.

A correlation exists between the occurrence of diabetes and BPA exposure. Levels are significantly higher in both borderline and diagnosed diabetic patients than in non-diabetics. Data also suggests that BPA increases the risk of cardiovascular disease and obesity. An analysis conducted in the U.S. between 2003 and 2008 with over 2,800 children aged 6 to 19 years revealed a significant association with obesity and urinary BPA concentrations.

BPA has thus been proposed as an environmental obesogen, contributing to worldwide obesity. Other studies conducted in the United States show a strong correlation between urinary BPA levels and cardiovascular disease.

Safety Classification

The National Toxicology Program shows "some concern" for the effects that BPA may have on the brain, prostate, and behavior in fetuses, infants, and children.

Health effects are more than likely related to recurrent exposure over time, and depend on the size and timing of the dose. Toxicity is generally associated with chronic exposure. The charts below can help determine where exposure to BPA may occur, and health concerns possibly related to BPA exposure. The final section provides resources and suggestions to reduce exposure.

OCCUPATIONS WHERE POSSIBLE BPA EXPOSURE MAY OCCUR:

Cashiers handling thermal receipt paper

Dentist or dental assistant

Employed in plastics industry or the manufacture of anything made from plastics

Employed in the paper industry

Recycling plant worker

POSSIBLE PERSONAL EXPOSURE TO BPA:

Consume lined canned foods (especially containing tomato products) or vegetable oils from plastic containers

Consume plastic-wrapped convenience foods

Consumption of fish or dairy products

Dental sealants, crown restorations

Drink bottled water or well water

Exposure to medical devices or procedures involving tubing or catheters, hemodialysis

Handling of thermal paper receipts, newspapers, magazines

Heat foods in plastic in microwave (frozen dinners, etc.), or microwave leftovers in to-go containers

Live near industries manufacturing plastics or products made from plastics

Living near a landfill or recycling plant

Recycled paper towels and toilet paper

Store food and beverages in plastic containers in hot garages

Use plastic cups, plates, tableware

Use plastic storage containers, plastic stretch wrap

POSSIBLE HEALTH CONCERNS ASSOCIATED WITH BPA EXPOSURE:

Abnormal liver enzymes

Alterations in thyroid and pituitary function

Asthma

Cardiovascular disease

Children's anxiety, hyperactivity, increased aggression, defiance, attention deficit

Diabetes, insulin resistance

Endometriosis, polycystic ovarian syndrome (PCOS)

Male genital abnormalities

Neurobehavioral complications

Obesity

Premature puberty

Prostate, testicular, and breast cancer

Recurrent miscarriages, premature labor, reduced birth weight

Reduced male fertility, declined sperm quality

EMPOWER YOURSELF

**WITH THESE ACTION STEPS AND BY USING THE
"RESOURCES AND SUGGESTIONS" THAT FOLLOW:**

Adhere to fish advisories

Avoid using beverages bottled in plastic and consider glass and stainless steel for food storage and beverages

Check for a supplier or manufacturer near your home

Check household products for BPA

Check if your canned goods are lined with BPA

Detoxify regularly

Do not handle receipts made with thermal paper, or wash your hands after handling

Explore safe options for storing leftovers, and for disposable dining ware

If you use well water, consider regular testing

Make sure employers adhere to occupational safety guidelines

Visit the Collaborative on Health and the Environment website for more information on BPA

Resources and Suggestions

Canned Foods

Reduce your use of canned foods or choose brands that are BPA free. The Environmental Working Group website updates information on BPA-lined canned food. It is available at: **http://www.ewg. org/research/bpa-canned-food.**

Databases for BPA

Check whether or not there is a chemical supplier or manufacturer near your home by visiting **http://www.thomasnet.com** and entering "Bisphenol A" into the search area. On the results page, you will have an opportunity to select your state to narrow down the search.

The National Library of Medicine, U.S. Department of Health and Human Services website, available at **https://hpd.nlm.nih.gov/**, lists products containing chemicals in the following categories: arts & crafts, auto products, commercial/institutional products, home office, home maintenance, inside the home, landscape/yard, personal care, pesticides, and pet care. One can do a "Quick Search" for the chemical name. On the Search Results page, select the "Primary Record" which will provide brand names of these household products.

The Collaborative on Health and the Environment website has several links of importance, such as "Environmental Risks" at **https://www.healthandenvironment.org/environmental-health/ environmental-risks/.** The 2011 Toxicant and Disease Database can be accessed at **https://www.healthandenvironment.org/our-work/**

toxicant-and-disease-database/, where one can search for either toxicants or diseases and disease categories associated with chemicals. as well as the link "Health, Diseases & Disabilities."

Fish Advisories

Adhere to fish advisories. While fish is considered a healthy protein containing essential fatty acids, frequent consumption increases risk, as seafood is a major contributor to dietary intake of BPA. The National Listing of Fish Advisories is available from the Environmental Protection Agency website at https://www.epa.gov/fish-tech/national-listing-fish-advisories-general-fact-sheet-2011, with more information on fish consumption at https://www.epa.gov/fish-tech.

Food Containers

Because heat increases the leaching of BPA into food from containers, don't microwave foods in plastic. While the FDA has banned BPA in baby bottles and sippy cups, Dr. Carl Baum at the Yale School of Medicine says some of the plasticizers replacing BPA may be even more dangerous for our children. Look for teethers and infant toys that are free of BPA. Dust often in the home and beware -- some plastics with the recycle code of 3 or 7 may still be made with BPA.

Whenever possible opt for stainless steel containers, porcelain, or glass. The leaching of BPA from plastics is enhanced when exposed to acidic or basic solutions and elevated temperatures. Coffee drinkers are advised not to use plastic coffee makers, and to take morning coffee to go in a stainless steel thermos. Using a French press to make coffee is recommended at home. If buying coffee at a café, take your own stainless steel thermos and avoid drinking out of the paper (or Styrofoam) cup, or through the plastic lid. Just one more reason not to smoke cigarettes? BPA is also present in cigarette filters, some containing up to 25% BPA.

Glass food storage containers are available at The Container Store, Crate and Barrel, Costco, Amazon, and at Bed, Bath, and Beyond, as well as other outlets. If these containers still use plastic lids, avoid contact by filling below the top so foods don't contact the lids or use a small plate to cover the dish. Also, avoid the use of plastic utensils and non-stick coated cookware, as well as the use of plastic stretch wrap when storing leftovers. Opt for tomato products that are available for purchase in glass and reuse the container afterward to store foods.

Explore other options for disposable cups, plates, and utensils. Eco Products features recyclable dining ware made from sugarcane and bamboo. You can access their website at: http://www.ecoprod uctsstore.com.

Alternative compostable and recyclable serving containers are available made with wheat straw fiber from World Centric Organization http://www.worldcentric.org/.

Unbleached paper snack and sandwich bags are available from the If You Care company at: https://www.ifyoucare.com/. Also, Etee Products can be found at https://www.shopetee.com.

OCCUPATIONAL EXPOSURE

Find out about worker rights and employer responsibilities regarding BPA by visiting Occupational Health and Safety Information at http://www.bisphenol-a.org/human/occsafety.html.

THERMAL RECEIPTS

The Environmental Working Group offers tips to reduce exposure from BPA in receipts and suggests not recycling thermal paper, letting a child hold or play with receipts, and washing hands before eating or preparing food after handling thermal papers. To check whether paper receipts are thermally treated, rub with a coin and if it does not discolor it is conventional paper. Electronic receipts are now being offered by many retailers. Other tips, along with research results, are available at http://www.ewg.org/research/bpa-in-store-receipts.

WATER TESTING

If you drink water from or bathe in well water, make sure to regularly test the quality of your water. The Centers for Disease Control and Prevention website has links to information on testing. It is available at: http://www.cdc.gov/healthywater/drinking/private/wells/.

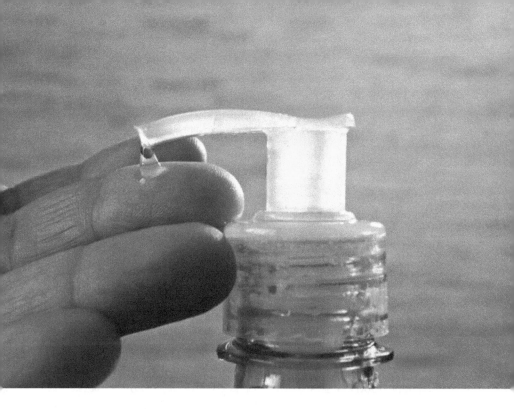

Chapter 7
SANITIZERS:
Triclosan

Triclosan was developed in 1964 as a component in detergent used for surgical scrubs. Because of triclosan's antimicrobial and antifungal properties, it is added to toothpaste, mouthwash, soap, shower gel, cosmetics, skin care lotions and cream, acne medication, deodorant, shampoo, wound disinfectants, ear plugs, combs, and hair brushes. Triclosan is used in the production of rubber materials, adhesives, caulks, grouts, paints, conveyor belts, ice-making machines, fire hoses, and used on heating and air conditioning coils. It is also added to food packaging to extend its shelf life by preventing micro-organism growth and preventing stains and odors. In 2009 Germany banned the use of triclosan as an additive used in the manufacture of plastics intended to contact food, followed by a ban in 2010 by the European Union. The US EPA and the FDA have rejected calls for a ban in the U.S.

Global production now exceeds 3 million pounds annually, of which 24% is produced in Europe. Approximately 900,000 pounds were used within the European Union in 2006. Although the Swedish government strongly discourages the use of antibacterial products, 25% of toothpastes in Sweden contain triclosan, translating to 4,000 pounds of triclosan consumed in toothpaste alone each year. Deodorants, soaps, and other personal care products account for another 700 pounds of the chemical in Sweden alone. Anti-microbial products were a $1.4 billion market in the U.S. in 2014.

Triclosan is found in household and industrial detergents, as well as in plastic cutting boards, coated metal knives, ceramic tiles, trash bags, food storage containers, cell phone covers, mulch, vacuum cleaners, food coolers, computer keyboards and mouse pads, mattresses, carpet, hot tubs, plastic lawn furniture, shower curtains, tents, awnings, garbage cans, sponges, brooms, baby changing stations, pacifiers, urinals and toilet bowls, protective sports gear, clothing, toys, and school supplies. Human exposure to triclosan occurs by ingestion and through skin absorption.

CONTAMINATED WATERS

Triclosan is washed down drains and enters both residential and commercial storm water systems. Since triclosan is only partially removed during wastewater treatment processes, it is detected in aquatic ecosystems. Sewage sludge is spread on land and triclosan leaches down through soil as it runs off into surface water from the fields. It has been detected as long as 266 days after application. Due to its bioaccumulative potential, levels of triclosan have been detected in a number of aquatic species, including elevated levels of triclosan reported in Rainbow trout in the Detroit River. Triclosan's estimated half-life in the aquatic environment is predicted to be 540 days, but some studies show measurable levels in the sediment core of lakes and estuaries, indicating a longer half-life.

Currently, there are no state or federal regulatory limits for triclosan in aquatic systems. In a U. S. Geological Survey study of 95 contaminants, triclosan was one of the most frequently detected and has some of the highest concentrations in U.S. streams. Triclosan has been detected in 75-100% of rivers, estuary waters and lakes in North American, Asia, Oceania, and Europe. High levels in South China were found in the Pearl River System. In the U.S. triclosan has been detected in New York's Hudson River Estuary, in Georgia, the Mississippi River, Key Largo Harbor, and in the Charleston, South Carolina Estuary.

INDOOR DUST

Triclosan also persists in indoor dust samples in private homes in considerable amounts and is likely associated with spills of personal care products, dead skin cells, treated textiles, and the use of household aerosol products containing triclosan.

PERSONAL CARE PRODUCTS

The United States Food and Drug Administration regulates the use of triclosan when incorporated into personal care products, laundry products, facial tissues, medical devices and antiseptics for wound care. The Environmental Protection Agency regulates triclosan when used as a pesticide, and also regulates its use as a material preservative. Since 1972, the use of triclosan has increased to the point that 75% of soaps contain the chemical. Because its use is not highly regulated, in December of 2013 the Food and Drug Administration began to further look into the safety of triclosan when they found that 76% of adults and children excrete it in their urine.

In a 2009 study, participants brushed their teeth twice daily for two weeks using triclosan-containing Colgate Total toothpaste. Because of its ability to alter the composition of oral flora, triclosan is added to toothpaste to reduce gingivitis and plaque. Blood samples collected prior to triclosan exposure were compared to the day following the termination of the study. Urine appears to be the main excretion pathway for triclosan and results indicated concentration levels were significantly higher at the end of the exposure period. Urinary excretion varies, but typically 24 to 83% of an oral dose is excreted within four days after exposure. Its half-life in the human body is relatively short at 65 hours in urine and would ordinarily be cleared from the body within that period of time. However in a study conducted in 2012, triclosan was detected in 10 out of 11 liver samples and 7 of 11 adipose tissue samples indicating a bioaccumulative effect.

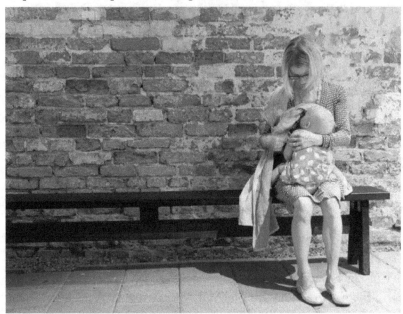

INFANTS AND CHILDREN

In humans, triclosan has been detected in urine, plasma, and breast milk, correlating with the pattern of consumer use. Of sixty-two breast milk samples tested from the Mother's Milk Banks in Texas and California, 81% samples contained triclosan. The detection of triclosan in breast milk raises the question as to the potential adverse effects to infants. Being exposed to a broad range of microbial agents early in life can suppress the development of the immune response, increasing a predisposition to allergic diseases. Urinary levels of triclosan and hay fever or allergy diagnosis in children have been positively associated. Triclosan was also found to weaken skeletal muscles and diminish the contractibility of cardiac muscles.

POTENTIALLY HORMONE DISRUPTING

Triclosan is a potential endocrine disruptor shown to decrease thyroid hormones (thyroxine and T3) while also altering testosterone and estrogen levels in animal studies. It's hypothesized that triclosan chemically mimics thyroid hormones and binds to receptor sites, blocking thyroid hormones made in the body. A study conducted on the North American bullfrog indicated that environmentally relevant levels of triclosan are capable of disrupting developmental processes that are dependent on thyroid hormones. Other studies demonstrate that triclosan decreases T3 and T4 levels in female rats. Decreases have also been observed in levels of hormones involved in reproduction including luteinizing hormone and follicle stimulating hormone, pregnenolone, and testosterone.

In pregnancy, studies have shown triclosan stimulated progesterone and estradiol secretion, while decreasing human chorionic gonadotropin. Triclosan could also potentially have a negative impact on the fetus and term of pregnancy. University of California Davis researchers found triclosan elevated calcium levels in cells, which could potentially affect neurological functioning and neurodevelopment. Sources of exposure for children under the age of 6 include household dust, breast milk, and mouthing of triclosan-treated plastics.

Childhood exposures remain a concern, due to the uncertainty about how triclosan may alter processes of growth and development. The largest study conducted on 623 Norwegian children between 2001 and 2004 indicated increased urinary levels were associated with asthma and rhinitis. Other potential health issues include antibiotic resistance, increasing rate of allergies, and skin irritation.

OBESITY AND THE GUT MICROBIOME

Several studies also suggest that endocrine disrupting compounds with antimicrobial properties can alter the bacterial flora in the human microbiome. The rapid rise in obesity parallels the use of triclosan, which has been shown to negatively modify the gut bacteria. Dysbiosis of the gut microbiome has attracted the attention of research and medicine in regards to its correlation to metabolic syndrome, mood disorders, cardiovascular disease, inflammatory bowel disorders, and obesity.

The European Union Scientific Committee on Consumer Products concluded that the maximum concentration of 0.3% is considered safe in personal care products, yet it's being questioned as to whether or not this amount is still safe due to concurrent exposures from multiple sources. Females were shown to have a significantly higher level of triclosan reflecting different hygiene habits than males, including their use of triclosan treated tampons and makeup.

Safety Classification

The Cancer Assessment Review Committee determined there is sufficient evidence for the tendency of triclosan to produce or tend to produce cancer of the liver in the mouse, although the U.S. EPA Final Guidance for Carcinogen Risk Assessment classified triclosan as "not likely to be carcinogenic to humans." The EPA is considering whether triclosan may be contaminated with dioxins as it reviews safety information.

Health effects are more than likely related to recurrent exposure over time, and depend on the size and timing of the dose. Toxicity is generally associated with chronic exposure. The charts below can help determine where exposure to triclosan may occur, and health concerns possibly related to triclosan exposure. The final section provides resources and suggestions to reduce exposure.

OCCUPATIONS WHERE POSSIBLE TRICLOSAN EXPOSURE MAY OCCUR:

Wastewater treatment, or with sewer sludge

Working with triclosan in manufacturing facilities

POSSIBLE PERSONAL EXPOSURE TO TRICLOSAN:

Consuming fish from triclosan-tainted waters, swimming in contaminated water

House dust

Triclosan-containing personal care products or pet products

Triclosan-containing products inside the home or for home maintenance

Using anti-bacterial soaps

Wearing anti-bacterial clothing

POSSIBLE HEALTH CONCERNS ASSOCIATED WITH TRICLOSAN EXPOSURE:

Altered gut bacteria

Asthma, rhinitis, skin irritations, hay fever, allergies

Imbalances in estrogens, progesterone, human chorionic gonadotropin

Neurological functioning and development issues

Weakened skeletal muscles, cardiac muscles

Adhere to fish advisories

Check for a supplier or manufacturer near your home

Check for triclosan-treated clothing

Check household products for triclosan

Consider an air filtration system

Detoxify regularly

Find triclosan-free personal care products

RESOURCES AND SUGGESTIONS

AIR AND SURFACE SANITIZING

It may be necessary to sanitize the air and surfaces in your home. Visit AirOasis at **http://www.airoasis.com/** to learn more about NASA developed technology.

DATABASES FOR TRICLOSAN

Check whether or not there is a chemical supplier or manufacturer near your home by visiting **http://www.thomasnet.com** and entering "triclosan" into the search area. On the results page, you will have an opportunity to select your state to narrow down the search.

The National Library of Medicine, U.S. Department of Health and Human Services website, available at https://hpd.nlm.nih.gov/, lists products containing chemicals in the following categories: arts & crafts, auto products, commercial/institutional products, home office, home maintenance, inside the home, landscape/yard, personal care, pesticides, and pet care. One can do a "Quick Search" for the chemical name. On the Search Results page, select the "Primary Record" which will provide brand names of these household products.

The FDA found that antibacterial products provide no benefit over soap and water, while the American Medical Association recommends antibacterial products not be used in the home as they may encourage bacterial resistance to antibiotics. The FDA published an online search database, the National Drug Code Directory, in 2009 to assist the public in determining which products contain questionable ingredients available at: https://www.accessdata.fda.gov/scripts/cder/ndc/index.cfm. When searching this link enter "Nonproprietary Name" for search type then enter triclosan for "name." Results show 500 personal care products containing this chemical (the website excludes housewares, shoes, and clothing.)

For information on occupational exposure to triclosan, visit the Santa Cruz Biotechnology datasheet at http://datasheets.scbt.com/sc-220326.pdf.

Fish Advisories

Adhere to fish advisories. The National Listing of Fish Advisories is available from the Environmental Protection Agency website at https://www.epa.gov/fish-tech/national-listing-fish-advisories-general-fact-sheet-2011, with more information on fish consumption at https://www.epa.gov/fish-tech.

Personal Care Products and Clothing

Avoiding products containing triclosan may be challenging because they are not always labeled as such, but rather mention "anti-bacterial." Check the labels when buying clothing, especially socks and shoes. Fiber and clothing that have triclosan incorporated into them may be referred to by the patented names of Microban, Ultra-Fresh, Monolith, Batonix, Sanitized, and Amicor. Triclosan containing personal care products include Colgate Total, Clearasil, Acne Wash, Murad Acne Complex Kit, and Old Spice High Endurance deodorant. Other brand names for triclosan include Aquasept, Spaoderm, Ster-Zac, Biofresh and Irgasan-DP300. As of 2014, Bath and Body Works removed triclosan from their hand soap collection.

You can also check personal care products for triclosan content at the website of the Environmental Working Group. Their Skin Deep database contains more than 73,000 products and can be accessed at http://www.ewg.org/skindeep/.

For more information on switching to triclosan-free products, contact Beyond Pesticides and Food & Water Watch at http://www. beyondpesticides.org/programs/antibacterials/triclosan. The website hosts a list of companies that have pledged to be triclosan free, as well as a sampling of products that contain triclosan or triclocarban. In December of 2010, a petition was filed by 82 environmental and public health groups, led by Beyond Pesticides and Food and Water Watch, to ban triclosan for non-medical use. A citizen petition was also submitted to the EPA in 2010 proposing a ban on triclosan in household products.

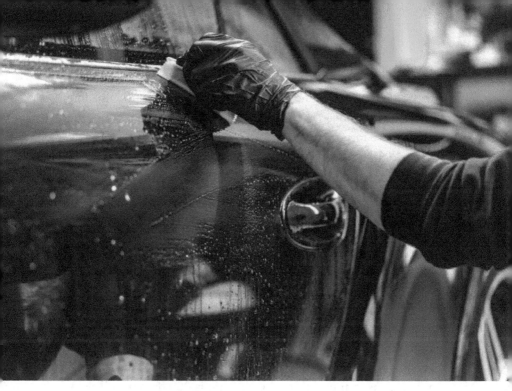

Chapter 8
SURFACTANTS:
4-NP

Four-nonylphenol (NP) is involved in the manufacture of nonyl-phenol ethoxylates (NPEs), which are surfactants that are mainly used for their emulsifying, wetting, and dispersing properties in cleaning and foaming agents. Industries use NP-containing products for institutional and industrial cleaning, agricultural pesticides, photographic film development, wall construction materials, paint production, correction fluids and inks, metal cleaning, vehicle cleaning, anti-static cleaners, leather degreasing, dyes, plastics, rubber, and wool scouring.

The electrical engineering industry utilizes NP-containing products in the manufacture of printed circuit boards and in dyes and chemical baths, as well as in cleaning products for electrical components. The veterinary industry uses NP-containing products in teat dips for controlling mastitis. These chemicals are also found in cosmetics, hair dyes, spermicides, detergents, food packaging, and are used in the formulation of paper products.

A 2010 estimate for the world's annual production of NPs is approximately 500 million pounds, with U.S. and Canadian demands estimated at 380 million pounds. The main source of NPs in the environment is its degradation in sewage treatment plants. In the mid-1990s Europe initiated the phasing out of this chemical, a policy followed ten years later by the United States.

ENVIRONMENTAL EXPOSURE

Surface water and sediments measured in the Great Lakes and along the Ohio River contain NP concentrations. NPs accumulate and persist in sewage sludge and river sediments, resulting from sewage treatment applications. Its half-life is 300 days in soil. NPs have been detected in ground water and river water, as well as in baby food and other food. Drinking water and food are thought to be the main sources of human exposure, although increased exposure has been shown to occur in children crawling on floors through carpet and floor cleaners containing NP products. NPs are a stabilizer used in plastics and may leach out of containers when coming into close contact with foods or fluids. Along with drinking water, NPs have been detected in cola soft drink samples and in milk and powdered milk samples.

DETECTED IN THE BODY

Research data shows urinary levels of NP has been detected in the urine of 51% of a sample of the general population in the U.S. Along with being detected in urine, NPs have also been detected in blood, breast milk, and umbilical cord blood. There is a positive correlation between fish and shellfish consumption and the levels of NPs in breast milk. Xenobiotic endocrine disruptors tend to accumulate in the body and are detectable in both adipose fat tissue and breast milk.

Noted Health Effects

A study conducted in 2013 showed NP exposure was associated with abnormal semen quality and male infertility, with impairment occurring at even low doses. Due to their ability to enhance inflammatory activities in the body, endocrine disruptors have also been identified as a risk factor in the development of allergic diseases by playing both an important role in triggering or exacerbating these diseases and influencing the onset, progression, and severity. NP exposure has also been linked to allergic lung inflammation. The highest concentrations of NPs in the body are found in the liver, followed by fat tissue and the brain.

Health effects are more than likely related to recurrent exposure over time, and depend on the size and timing of the dose. Toxicity is generally associated with chronic exposure. The charts below can help determine where exposure to NPs may occur, and health concerns possibly related to NP exposure. The final section provides resources and suggestions to reduce exposure.

OCCUPATIONS WHERE POSSIBLE NP EXPOSURE MAY OCCUR:

Employed where NPs are manufactured or used

Industrial and institutional cleaning

Photographic film developing

Work in electrical engineering industry, veterinary field, or sewage treatment

POSSIBLE PERSONAL EXPOSURE TO NPS:

Amateur photographic film developing

Carpet and floors cleaned with NP-containing products

Cosmetic use, hair dyes, spermicides

Detergents, cleaning products

Fish and shellfish consumption

Living near a textile factory that uses NPs

POSSIBLE HEALTH CONCERNS ASSOCIATED WITH NP EXPOSURE:

Abnormal semen quality, male infertility

Allergic diseases

Premature puberty

EMPOWER YOURSELF

WITH THESE ACTION STEPS AND BY USING THE "RESOURCES AND SUGGESTIONS" THAT FOLLOW

Adhere to fish advisories

Check for a supplier or manufacturer near your home

Check products that contain nonylphenol

Know your rights when occupationally exposed

DATABASES FOR NONYLPHENOL

Check whether or not there is a chemical supplier or manufacturer near your home by visiting **http://www.thomasnet.com** and entering "nonylphenol" into the search area. On the results page, you will have an opportunity to select your state to narrow down the search.

The National Library of Medicine, U.S. Department of Health and Human Services website, available at **https://hpd.nlm.nih.gov/**, lists products containing chemicals in the following categories: arts & crafts, auto products, commercial/institutional products, home office, home maintenance, inside the home, landscape/yard, personal care, pesticides, and pet care. One can do a "Quick Search" for the chemical name. On the Search Results page, select the "Primary Record" which will provide brand names of these household products.

If the product is not on the list, check the safety by visiting the Material Safety Data Sheet at **http://msds.com/**.

FISH ADVISORIES

For fish consumption advisories, visit the Environmental Protection Agency's website: **https://www.epa.gov/fish-tech**.

OCCUPATIONAL EXPOSURE

The United States Department of Labor website for Occupational Safety and Health Administration contains information on worker's rights. It is available at **https://www.osha.gov/workers/index.html**.

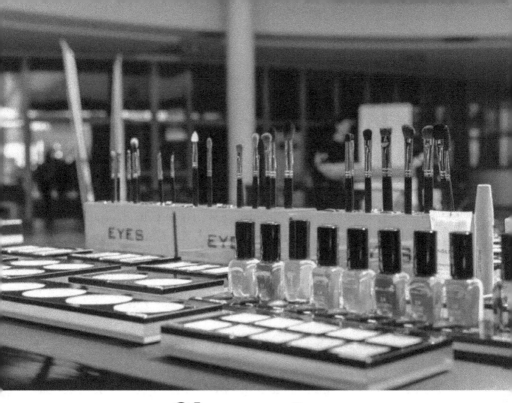

Chapter 9
ANTIBACTERIALS IN PERSONAL CARE PRODUCTS:
Parabens

Parabens are used as an antimicrobial preservative in a wide range of consumer products including pharmaceuticals, medical products, personal care products, and as a preservative in paper products. Its metabolites include methylparaben, propylparaben, butylparaben, ethylparaben, and isobutylparaben. The majority of parabens are produced in China, with production of each paraben reported to be 20 million pounds per year. Exposure to parabens occurs orally, topically, and a small amount is through inhalation. Results from the 2006 NHANES (National Health and Nutrition Examination Survey) report indicates that propylparaben and methylparaben are detected in approximately 93% and 99% of human tissue samples, respectively.

Paraben metabolites have been measured in fruits and vegetables, and in medication. Globally parabens have been detected in soil, sediment, wastewaters and in surface waters in Canada, India, Japan, China, South Korea, Spain, Switzerland, the United Kingdom, and the United States. In 2010 parabens were detected in 44% of cosmetic products and in 8% of detergents, with methylparaben and propylparaben heading the list.

PERSONAL CARE PRODUCTS

Researchers have suggested that dermal exposure to parabens can be biologically substantial in just a single application of lotion to the chest and breast area, causing significant estrogenic exposure to tissues. Limits have been set on the paraben content allowed in personal care products; however, consumers typically do not use just one product on a daily basis so limits to exposure are often exceeded. The measurement of parabens detected in humans demonstrates that these compounds escape metabolism when applied dermally, as opposed to undergoing liver and intestinal metabolic processes when exposed orally, thus allowing for greater internal exposure.

When low-level paraben-containing personal care products are left on the skin for continuous exposure over the long term, such as deodorant, it can result in an accumulation in the underlying tissues. Studies in 2007 and 2008 showed that parabens were detected in the bloodstream within one hour of dermal application, again escaping metabolic breakdown. Long-term exposure to parabens have been linked to metastatic processes. Dermal exposure to parabens from personal care products that are used in the breast region and under the arm enter human tissue intact and bind to estrogen receptors. Parabens have been detected in the amniotic fluid and urine of pregnant women, with both propylparaben and methylparaben found in

99% of samples.

The European Union's Scientific Committee on Consumer Safety (SCCS) suggests that sunscreen should not be applied to infants up to 6 months of age, but rather protecting them from sunlight with adequate clothing and shade.

Hormone Disrupting

Parabens are endocrine disrupting compounds that have been shown to stimulate the growth of breast cancer cells. First detected in breast tumor tissues in 2004, studies that followed detected parabens in seminal fluid, blood, breast milk, and placental tissue tested around the world. With the incidence of breast cancer increasing in postmenopausal women, it has been suggested that when ovarian production of estrogen drops, exogenous estrogens fuel the receptors sites and influence the expression of cells. In 2012 researchers took 160 tissue samples from four locations in the breast and armpit from 40 breast cancer patients undergoing mastectomies. One or more paraben was found in 99% of samples and 60% contained all five parabens measured, with methylparaben constituting 60% of the content followed by propylparaben at 13%, butylparaben at 11%, and ethylparaben at 10% of the total composition. Of all parabens, in Switzerland methylparaben was detected at the highest level in human milk, followed by ethylparaben and propylparaben.

Women show a three to four-fold increased level of parabens in urine than men, resulting from their higher use of personal care products. Adolescent girls between the ages of 12 and 16 years can have an even higher exposure than adult women. African Americans showed more than three times higher rates of exposure than Caucasians, however this may be attributable to either pharmaceutical use or personal care product use. Of the five common parabens showing endocrine disrupting properties, isobutylparaben binds most strongly to estrogen receptor sites followed by butylparaben, propylparaben, ethylparaben, and then methylparaben. While their binding ability is considered weaker than estrogens made in the body, their increase in concentration can have the same level of binding as the stronger estradiol.

Research conducted at Massachusetts General Hospital's Fertility Center suggests that exposure to propylparaben may contribute to ovarian aging and diminished ovarian function in women seeking treatment for infertility. Parabens have also been reported to cause beta cell dysfunction, affecting insulin secretion following spikes in blood glucose concentrations. They have also been shown to be anti-androgenic, decreasing sperm function and inhibiting testosterone.

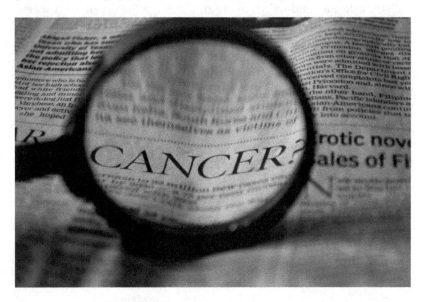

Breast Cancer

Distribution of parabens was also studied. A disproportionate increase in breast cancer was found in the upper outer quarter of the breast (i.e. near the armpit), suggesting the deposit of parabens in the area resulted from application of personal care products in that region. It's interesting to note that seven out of 40 women reported never using deodorant and yet they had measurable amounts of parabens in that region, suggesting parabens can migrate from one area to another and that there are other environmental sources of exposure. In the United Kingdom, breast cancers located in the upper outer area of the breast now exceed 50%. Levels of parabens found in tissue have concentrations that result in environmental impacts. It has been proposed that chemicals may accumulate in this area of the breast due to lymphatic or local circulatory mechanisms that have yet to be determined. While there may not be ample evidence that parabens cause breast cancer, there are signs of concern indicating that these compounds are not safe.

In 2011 Denmark notified the SCCS that it banned propylparaben and butylparaben in products for children under the age of three, citing reproductive toxicity and adverse effects on male reproductive endpoints. Also suggested was to ban the use of paraben-containing products for infants around the diaper region. It's been proposed in research that the estrogenic burden of parabens may exceed the action of estradiol in children, and that long-term low-level exposures beginning so early in life may be priming them for later effects. It's also been proposed that methylparaben is more suitable as a rinse off product rather than a leave-on and that any skin with a damaged barrier is unsuitable for application of paraben-containing personal care products, while emphasizing that shaving armpits and facial hair can enhance absorption when skin is nicked.

Safety Classification

In 2011 parabens were added to the SIN (Substitute It Now) list of Sweden's International Chemical Secretariat. The US Food and Drug Administration determined that parabens are safe for use in cosmetics, following an *industry-led review* in 2006. As a result, parabens are not regulated in the United States. The World Health Organization has excluded propylparaben and butylparaben from use as food additives. Data suggests some degree of bioaccumulation of parabens during life, but it has yet to be determined.

Health effects are more than likely related to recurrent exposure over time, and depend on the size and timing of the dose. Toxicity is generally associated with chronic exposure. The charts below can help determine where exposure to parabens may occur, and health concerns possibly related to paraben exposure. The final section provides resources and suggestions to reduce exposure.

OCCUPATIONS WHERE POSSIBLE PARABEN EXPOSURE MAY OCCUR:

Work in manufacturing where parabens are used: personal care products industry, pet products, air fresheners, preservatives in foods

POSSIBLE PERSONAL EXPOSURE TO PARABENS:

Consuming medication with parabens listed as an ingredient

Consumption of contaminated fish

Using personal care products, pet products, or products inside the home containing parabens

POSSIBLE HEALTH CONCERNS ASSOCIATED WITH PARABEN EXPOSURE:

Breast cancer

Diabetes and insulin related disorders

Infertility and reproductive dysfunction in males and females

Low testosterone in males, decreased sperm functioning

Premature menopause

WITH THESE ACTION STEPS AND BY USING THE
"RESOURCES AND SUGGESTIONS" THAT FOLLOW

Adhere to fish advisories

Check household products for parabens

Check medications for parabens

Check personal care products for parabens

Detoxify regularly

Visit ChemSec's website for more information on producers of hazardous chemicals in Europe

RESOURCES AND SUGGESTIONS:

DATABASE FOR PARABENS

The National Library of Medicine, U.S. Department of Health and Human Services website, available at **https://hpd.nlm.nih.gov/**, lists products containing chemicals in the following categories: arts & crafts, auto products, commercial/institutional products, home office, home maintenance, inside the home, landscape/yard, personal care, pesticides, and pet care. One can do a "Quick Search" for the chemical name. On the Search Results page, select the "Primary Record" which will provide brand names of these household products.

To search for more information on hazardous chemicals, visit the ChemSec SIN list at **http://chemsec.org/business-tool/sin-list/**

FISH ADVISORIES

Adhere to fish advisories and limit fatty fish intake. The National

---

Listing of Fish Advisories is available from the Environmental Protection Agency website at **https://www.epa.gov/fish-tech/national-listing-fish-advisories-general-fact-sheet-2011**, with more information on fish consumption at **https://www.epa.gov/fish-tech**.

MEDICATIONS WITH METHYLPARABEN

Top medications containing methylparaben can be searched at: https://www.drugs.com/inactive/methylparaben-290.html

Personal Care Products

Products containing parabens include: body lotions, face creams and facial cleansing products, hand soap, shower bathing gels, toothpastes, make up, sunscreen, hair removers, shampoos, hair conditioners, shaving creams and after-shave products, diaper rash ointments, hair coloring, pet personal products, antibacterial soaps, stain removers, foundation, powder, blush, mascara, eye pencils, lip color, eye shadows, cleansing cloths, baby lotions, styling products, antiperspirants, deodorants, lice treatment, and others.

The Environmental Working Group's website, EWG's Skin Deep, allows users to search for a specific personal product out of their database of nearly 73,000 specific products. Once the exact product has been located, the results will provide ingredient concerns rated as low, moderate, or high. Also included is the specific concern as it relates to cancer, developmental and reproductive toxicity, allergies and immunotoxicity, along with its overall hazard. The website is available at: http://www.ewg.org/skindeep/. Search the app store for EWG Healthy Living to access information on your smart phone or iPad. It also has a bar code reader for ease of use in determining safe products while shopping. You simply allow access to your camera by the app.

The Breast Cancer Action website provides a list of paraben-free cosmetic companies. It is available at http://www.bcaction.org/our-take-on-breast-cancer/environment/safe-cosmetics/paraben-free-cosmetics/.

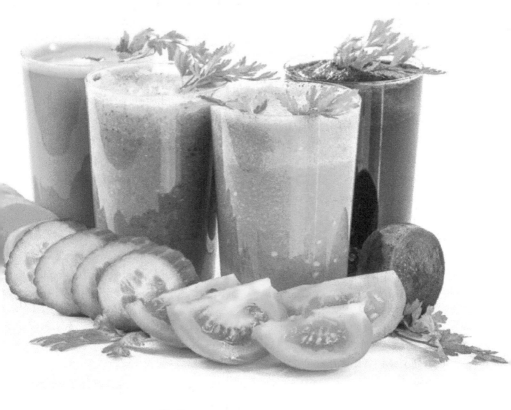

Chapter 10
DETOXIFICATION

Although thousands of studies have analyzed how exposure to environmental toxicants occurs in humans, little attention has been paid to addressing therapeutic interventions that effectively remove these chemicals from the body. The World Health Organization's (WHO) data from 2008 suggests that 7.6 million cancer deaths annually can be attributed to factors that include environmental toxins, estimating that number will reach 11.4 million in 2030. In 2009 WHO data estimated 40% of human deaths around the world each year can be attributed to environmental factors. Those groups at the highest level of exposure include infants, children, the elderly and those employed in industry. Pregnant and lactating women are also vulnerable groups.

Copious amounts of scientific literature exist that correlate the erosion of health with the body's bioaccumulation of toxicants, but the field of environmental health sciences is still in its infancy. One of the challenges to research is that humans aren't exposed to just a single chemical, but rather mixtures of pollutants from multiple chemical classes and sources. For example, the half-life of DDT in the body is 8 years. If one gram were absorbed into fat stores in 1972, there would still be .12 grams in body fat in 1996 and .04 grams in 2004 – that's if the person was never exposed to additional DDT during those periods. And that's just *one* chemical. With millions of chemical compounds existing around the globe, regulatory codes can monitor only a fraction of them so exposure continues to both humans and the environment.

PRENATAL PLANNING

It's critical that when *planning* a family young couples take detoxification into serious consideration. Environmental contaminants in mothers are transferred during pregnancy and lactation to offspring. In 2004 testing revealed that the average number of chemicals found in umbilical cord blood registered at 287 chemicals, meaning children begin their lives in the womb exposed to an average of 180 toxicants that are considered carcinogenic to humans, 208 that cause abnormal development in laboratory animals and 217 that are toxic to the brain and nervous system. After the womb children continue to have unique pathways of exposure differing from adults: they drink breast milk or formula, use hand-to and object-to-mouth exploration, they live lower to the ground and experience different breathing zones. In addition, their ability to metabolize, detoxify and excrete toxins is still developing.

An estimated 2,000 new chemicals are being introduced into consumer products and foods each year in the United States with over 83,000 chemicals currently being released into the environment worldwide. The Pediatric Academic Societies speculate that low levels of toxic chemicals may be impacting the functioning of the current generation, while other medical bodies and researchers conclude exposure may also be affecting future generations beyond just the current.

Toxicant Induced Loss of Tolerance

Chemical sensitivities, food intolerances, and acquired allergies may develop in response to toxicant exposure resulting in reactions to common food incitants, such as: gluten, casein, corn, soy, MSG (monosodium glutamate), artificial sweeteners and colors, nuts, yeast, eggs, and foods in the nightshade family (tomatoes, potatoes, eggplant, and peppers.) This condition has been termed TILT, an acronym for toxicant induced loss of tolerance. Avoiding these foods and undergoing detoxification can help improve symptoms. Any number of the following symptoms could be indicative of a need to enhance the body's natural detoxification systems:

Bad breath and body odor

Bloating and gas

Fatigue with sleep disruption and brain fog

Fluid retention and excess weight

Headaches with neck and shoulder pain

Heartburn

Infertility and low interest in sex

Irritable bowel, foul - smelling stools, and dark urine

Mood disturbance, especially depression, anxiety, fear, and anger

Muscle aches and joint pain

Premature aging and weakness

Rashes and canker sores

Recurrent colds, and persistent infections

Sinus congestion, dark circles under the eyes, and post-nasal drip

Weight changes and loss of muscle tone

The Detoxification Process

The liver is the key organ of detoxification in the body, but considerable amounts of detoxification can also occur in the brain, lungs, kidneys, and intestines. If the toxicant is lipid-soluble, detoxification will typically begin with transforming the fat-soluble compound into a water-soluble compound through Phase I enzymes in the liver. This reaction helps prepare it for excretion from the body. Yet, Phase I transformation doesn't always sufficiently render the toxin soluble enough to complete the excretion pathway, so Phase II enzymes modify the compound to both increase its solubility and reduce its toxicity.

A balance between Phase I and Phase II processes must be struck. Following Phase I metabolism, the original toxicants can potentially be more destructive than before the conversion and if Phase II enzymes are not able to neutralize them as rapidly as they are formed, the risk of cellular damage increases or a healing crisis may occur. A healing crisis is a temporary worsening of symptoms that sometimes occurs during detoxification.

Common symptoms of a healing crisis can include:

Bloating

Body aches

Cramping

Diarrhea

Fatigue

Headache

Lightheadedness

Mood changes

Weakness

However, these symptoms can also develop as withdrawal symptoms from avoiding caffeine, alcohol, sugar, and nicotine during detoxification. It's typically best to continue with the detoxification process when symptoms occur, being sure to rule out electrolyte imbalances, low fluid intake, and low blood sugar.

Phase III transporters, present in many tissues throughout the body, move Phase II products out of the cells by transporting them through bile secretions from the gallbladder into the intestines or through the bloodstream to the kidneys for excretion. The kidneys will further process the chemicals by filtering them and then excreting them in urine. Typically, water soluble metabolites are eliminated in the urine, and fat soluble metabolites are excreted through feces.

Toxicants are transported to the small intestines where they can enter cells lining the intestinal lumen. If they are reabsorbed back into the blood they return to the liver, resulting in a recycling of toxicants. This requires more energy and nutrients for the liver, it prolongs the half-life of the chemical compound, and the kidneys must reabsorb the toxicant as it filters the blood, resulting in persistent exposures.

THE GUT MICROBIOME

Research has shown that restoration of the damaged microbial environment in the intestinal flora can facilitate the removal of certain toxicants. Calcium D-glucarate may improve the intestinal bacterial balance, as can modified citrus pectin (MCP). Studies have shown that consuming pectin may play an important role in cleaning the digestive tract. It can reduce pathogenic bacteria and stimulate the growth of healthy bacterial strains such as Bifidobacteria and Lactobacillus, rendering it useful for long-term detoxification without side effects.

While toxins are in transit through the gastrointestinal tract, kaolin and bentonite clays and activated charcoal can prevent adhesion of the toxicants to the surface of the gut or to other molecules in the gut. Beneficial colonic microflora has a similar effect. Colonic irrigations have been used to reduce body burdens of chlorinated pesticides and PCBs, as has sauna therapy, and these protocols might be valuable for chronically ill patients experiencing weight loss in order to reduce toxic levels in the blood.

Assisting Detoxification Phases

If there is a deficiency in these nutrients or a high carbohydrate diet that is low in protein, Phase I enzymes are decreased and metabolic clearance is slowed. In animals, calcium deprivation increased the absorption of cadmium and lead. Phase I detoxification activity can be increased with:

Minerals calcium, magnesium, iron, zinc, copper, selenium

Protein

Vitamins A, B2, B3, folate, C, E

It is important to note that a decrease in Phase II enzyme activity is associated with aging. Phase II enzymes require:

Foods containing the amino acids l-methionine
and l-cysteine

Glutathione

SAMe

Vitamins B2, B3, B5, B6, B12

While grapefruit has been well confirmed in its ability to increase
Phase II enzymatic activity while slowing Phase I activities, (suggesting its avoidance while taking prescription drugs), the following
plants and nutrients can increase both Phase I and Phase II enzymatic activities:

Alpha lipoic acid

Capsicum

Chlorophyll

Citrus oil

Cruciferous vegetables

Curcumin

Garlic

Gingko biloba

Glutathione

Green tea

Hops

Horseradish

Indole-3-carbinol

Lycopene

Milk thistle

N-acetyl cysteine (NAC)

Olives

Probiotics

Quercetin

Resveratrol

Rutin

As Phase III transporters move Phase II products out of the cell, they can decrease the effectiveness of certain pharmaceutical therapies by increasing clearance of the drug, something that can be problematic with chemotherapy or other medications. Constituents in apple and broccoli stimulate Phase III, while curcumin, milk thistle, and resveratrol decrease its activity.

Secreted from the gallbladder, bile is an important transporter of toxins from the body by moving them out of the liver and into the intestines for elimination. Aside from pharmaceutical options, artichoke can both protect the liver and stimulate bile flow. Other plants shown to enhance bile flow include dandelion, fennel, yarrow, garlic, curry, ginger, cumin, mustard leaf, and andrographis - an herbaceous plant native to India.

Weight Loss and the Obesity Paradox

Due to their affinity to accumulate in fat tissue, toxicants are released from storage during rigorous exercise, illness, fasting, or weight loss. When this occurs an increase in concentration develops in the blood and then re-enters circulation, having the ability to reach critical organs for deposition. Fifteen weeks after bariatric surgery individuals showed an increase in the concentrations of several persistent organic pollutants.

In obese elderly participants with low persistent organic pollutant concentrations, mortality increased with fat mass. However, obese individuals with high levels of toxic concentrations showed lower mortality. The phenomenon of the obesity paradox can be explained in that fat provides a "safe" storage for toxic chemicals. Some pollutants have half-lives from several years to a decade and the negative health effects of high fat mass may be overshadowed by the benefit it provides in protecting the body from the harmful effects of stored pollutants, leading to questions regarding the safety of weight loss among obese patients with chronic diseases. Recall, however, that obesity itself can increase the half-lives of toxicants.

Exercise and Sweating Assists Detoxification

Exercise stimulates liver detoxification enzymes and promotes excretion through the kidneys and skin. It's recommended that glutathione be administered in creams, intravenously, nebulized, or in a liposomal preparation to increase its bioavailability. Glutathione enhancers, along with sauna therapy and vigorous exercise, can facilitate the movement of toxicants from fat storage. N-acetylcysteine, MSM (methylsulfonylmethane) and l-taurine support glutathione synthesis, as do sulfur-containing foods such as eggs, brassicas and alliums, and DMSA (dimercaptosuccinic acid) supplementation. Along with l-taurine, the amino acids l-glycine and l-glutamine are also involved in toxicant elimination.

As toxicants are mobilized from fat storage sites, the skin can enhance detoxification through sweating. Various researchers have confirmed that body burdens are reduced with sweating during exercise or by sitting in a sauna. The skin is a significant organ of detoxification and numerous toxicants can be excreted through perspiration, some of which were never detected in serum during clinical studies.

In Scandinavian countries the use of saunas has been a constant practice for hundreds of years. Nearly two million saunas are located in Finland for a population of just 5.3 million people. Dr. William Rea, Director of the Environmental Health Center in Dallas, Texas documents the results of sauna usage in his patients undergoing detoxification. His comprehensive program involves radiant-heat sauna therapy with a temperature between 140 and 160 degrees, followed by oral vitamins, minerals, and amino acids, and an IV of vitamin C.

Naturopathic physician Dr. Walter Crinnion has utilized sauna therapy with his patients for 20 years in the Seattle area. He reveals that following a comprehensive protocol that includes saunas, it was not unusual for the smell of chemicals to exude from patients. Over 84% of those suffering from multiple chemical sensitivities and autoimmune disorders reported good to great improvement after following his detoxification program.

Dry skin brushing not only exfoliates dead cells from the skin, it is also said to be effective at stimulating the lymphatic system. Dry skin brushing became popular in the early 1940s when Swedish naturopath Paavo Airola and Californian chiropractor Bernard Jensen both advocated the practice. Dry skin brushes have been sold in health food stores for over 70 years. Thirty-minute baths using sea salt or Kosher salt and baking soda have been said to also help to draw toxins through the skin.

NUTRITION

In supporting natural detoxification pathways, several foods have also been proposed that reduce absorption and reabsorption of toxins including insoluble fiber, chlorella, cilantro, sulphur containing amino acids (taurine and methionine), and sulphur-rich foods in the brassica and allium family, such as:

Arugula

Bok choy

Broccoli

Brussels sprouts

Cabbage

Cauliflower

Chinese cabbage

Chives

Collard greens

Garlic

Horseradish

Kale

Kohlrabi

Leeks

Mustard greens

Onions

Radishes

Rutabaga

Scallions

Shallots

Turnips

Wasabi

Watercress

While a poor nutritional state can worsen toxicity in the body, a high nutritional status that includes calcium, zinc, iron, selenium, folate, and omega-3 fatty acids has been shown to both reduce absorption and facilitate the excretion of persistent organic pollutants, as has insoluble fiber and plant foods such as turmeric, alliums, chlorella, algae, and quercitin. Diets rich in omega-3 fatty acids and antioxidants also have been shown to reduce toxicant-induced inflammation. The antioxidant resveratrol can limit proinflammatory processes in the body and protect cells from damaging free radical scavengers. For a list of foods high in specific nutrients, such as resveratrol, visit the World's Healthiest Foods website at **http://www.whfoods.com/** and enter the name of the food in the search bar.

Therapies that inhibit dietary fat absorption are discussed in literature, having been found to enhance fecal excretion of toxicants that dissolve in fat. Pharmaceutical drugs Olestra and Orlistat have been shown to be effective in enhancing excretion of several chemicals, such as dioxins, PCBs, and hexachlorobenzene. Natural lipase inhibitors include guar gum, psyllium hulls, and lecithin. Lipase inhibitors decrease the gastrointestinal absorption of fat. Research has suggested that pepsin and bovine or porcine bile supplementation may increase the mobilization and solubility of persistent organic pollutants and enhance their elimination.

Japanese studies show the daily use of rice bran fiber and chlorophyll increases the clearance of PCBs and dioxins. Matcha green tea showed an increased excretion of PCBs by 4.4 times. White teas have also shown similar effects in reducing the total body burden, however it has been suggested that steeping tea for longer than 3 minutes is not advisable due to the increase in detectable levels of heavy metals. Hemicellulose fibers in wheat bran, nuts, and legumes have an affinity for organic pollutants, inhibiting their absorption. Lignans in flax and sesame seeds show even higher sorptive properties, especially with pesticides that dissolve in fats. Korean red ginseng significantly decreased urinary BPA levels from the 4th day of treatment in one clinical study, and vitamin E has been shown to restore antioxidant activities in the liver of rats exposed to atrazine.

Consumption of fresh water algae Chlorella resulted in a significant reduction of dioxin levels in breast milk in Japanese women, and reduced the half-life of the persistent organic pollutant chlordecone. Nori seaweed has been shown to prevent the absorption of dioxins, while Wakame seaweed increased excretion by two times. Bentonite clay and psyllium husks may decrease the re-uptake of some compounds and are being studied as detoxifying agents in the body. Animal studies show the ingestion of zeolite minerals bind toxins for excretion.

DETOXIFICATION PROGRAMS

The website for the University of Wisconsin's Integrative Medicine department, under the direction of Dr. David Rakel, offers the pdf file "Detoxification to Promote Health: A 7-Day Program" available at http://www.fammed.wisc.edu/sites/default/files//webfm-uploads/documents/outreach/im/handout_detoxplan.pdf. The document includes suggestions for fasting and skin brushing, and two variations of a 7-day detox including a recipe for a "Superfoods Detox Broth." It's very similar to the Vital Broth recipe included in Dr. Bernard Jensen's 1984 publication "*Vital Foods for Total Health*" which features his "Eleven-Day Elimination Diet."

Included in the University's program is the suggested use of hydrolyzed whey protein powder to assist the liver in making more glutathione for detoxification, along with pectasol powder (MCP), milk thistle, dandelion, turmeric, probiotics, and a multivitamin, with a note to include activated charcoal or bentonite clay on fasting days.

The protein from whey is considered to be better assimilated than other protein in cases of low hydrochloric acid levels.

Studies have shown that chlorophyll promotes a strong immune response with a scientific basis as being useful for bowel disease and a hyper immune system response. N-acetyl-cysteine (NAC) was shown to enhance mobilization of toxicants from tissue storage sites and increase their rate of elimination. NAC was also able to reduce and remove arsenic from organs. Bentonite clay and activated charcoal can decrease the re-uptake and interrupt the recirculation of some toxicants in the body by absorbing them. Algin and chlorella are gaining attention as having the potential to absorb heavy metals and have been used successfully to reduce lead and mercury in case studies, while malic acid appears to assist with the removal of aluminum. Cilantro has been reported to enhance mercury excretion following dental amalgam removal and decrease lead absorption in the bones of animals. Probiotics restore the damaged germ environment in the intestinal flora, with emerging evidence indicating they facilitate gastrointestinal excretion of selected toxicants.

HERBS COMMONLY USED FOR DETOXIFICATION

In the early 1930s John R. Christopher, an herbalist from Salt Lake City, worked with some of the last remaining Native American medicine men in the Western United States. Like the Scandinavians, Native American Indians believed in the value of sweating. Sage tea was known to promote perspiration and was drank as a hot tea during most illnesses. But the medicinal use of herbs doesn't begin there. In fact, the oldest written evidence of plants being used as medicine was found on a 5,000-year-old clay slab in India, referencing over 250 plants. A Chinese book written around 2500 BC outlines the medicinal use of 365 plants. Herbs can support the cleansing and removal of waste, and combining herbs can provide a synergistic effect to help activate the body's cleansing abilities and enhance the elimination of toxic accumulation.

The horticulture schools of Purdue University at **https://hort.pur due.edu/ newcrop/Indices/index_ab.html** hosts a plethora of information on the history and use of medicinal herbs, as does the website https://botanical.com/botanical/mgmh/comindxa.html.

The following plants are well known in herbal healing for their detoxification properties, usefulness in strengthening the organs of detoxification, and in providing relief during a healing crisis. Most often they are used in combination.

Aloe – used for thousands of years for constipation, one of the most frequently prescribed herbs throughout most of the 18th and 19th centuries and remains one of the most commonly used herbs in the United States today

Buckthorn – laxative properties

Burdock root – blood purifier, diuretic, high in antioxidants, aids the skin

Capsicum – anti-bacterial effects, used as food and medicine for over 9,000 years

Cascara sagrada – promotes peristalsis (wavelike movement in the gut)

Couch grass – diuretic demulcent

Dandelion root – detoxify liver and gallbladder, aid in kidney function, used for diarrhea

Fenugreek – soothes inflamed conditions of the stomach and intestines

Ginger – used for over 2,000 years for nausea, liver protective, anti-spasmodic, improves tone of intestinal muscles, anti-diar-rheal

Grapefruit essential oil – anti-fungal, diuretic, improves lymphatic circulation

Lemon essential oil – anti-microbial, anti-viral, anti-hepatotoxic (liver toxicity) activities, diuretic properties

Licorice –soothing and coating agent, diuretic, expectorant, laxative

Marshmallow – gel forming to coat stomach and reduce irritation, anti-inflammatory, used for over 2,000 years as both a medicine and a food

Milk thistle – protect the liver from toxins, helps liver repair itself

Oregon grape – improves digestion and absorption

Peppermint essential oil – used for allaying headache, vomiting, nausea, with antibacterial, antiviral, and antifungal properties

Psyllium –softens stool, fermenting plant

Red clover – anti-fungal, expectorant, anti-spasmodic, blood purifier, diuretic

Sarsaparilla – rehydrate the body, anti-microbial, aids liver, anti-diarrheal

Turkey rhubarb – astringent action, helpful in cases of diarrhea

Yellow dock – blood purifier, tonic to the stomach

In addition, one can search for information on herbs and supplements at the National Institutes of Health National Center for Complementary and Integrative Health at **https://nccih.nih.gov/health/ atoz.htm,** with additional information on herbs on the Memorial Sloan Kettering Cancer Center website **https://www.mskcc.org/ cancer-care/diagnosis-treatment/symptom-management/integra tive-medicine/herbs/search.**

Herbal Medicine Contraindications

It's extremely important to remember that there are multiple contraindications to be aware of when using herbs and supplements in conjunction with pharmaceutical medication. For instance, it is well understood that grapefruit intake should be avoided when taking certain medications because of its enzyme binding ability, meaning the medication can pass through the body more quickly than intended. Statin drugs, calcium channel blockers, and psychiatric medications are some of the most common drugs that interact with grapefruit. The science-based *Natural Medicines Comprehensive Database* allows one to search for any natural product and drug interaction, the nutrient depletion caused by a medication, a natural product's effectiveness, and includes several other reports and series. It is available in book form or by electronic subscription at **http://naturaldatabase.thera peuticresearch.com/home.aspx?cs=&s=ND**. One can also refer to the booklet, *"Plant Medicine Safety"* by this author.

Contaminated vs. Quality Supplements

In addition, recall that herbs and supplements can become contaminated by absorbing toxic elements from the soil and their environment, especially if not analyzed for purity before going into the marketplace. The U.S. Food and Drug Administration's website hosts recall information on dietary supplements and foods **http://www. fda.gov/food/recallsoutbreaksemergencies/recalls/default.htm,** but also check with NSF International for companies in compliance with Good Manufacturing Processes **http://info.nsf.org/Certified/GMP/**.

Human Toxicant Testing

Human biomonitoring is a simple tool that assesses exposure to pollutants and can monitor how well human detoxification programs are working. Human biomonitoring values from Germany's main environmental protection agency, the German Human Biomonitoring Commission, are available for more than 130 chemical constituents at this time (http://www.umweltbundesamt.de/en/topics/chemicals.) The Israel Ministry of Health also measures select occupational groups for environmental toxicants through its National Biomonitoring Study.

Analyzing both urine and blood serum can determine biomarkers for pesticides, PCBs, flame retardants, and many other chemicals. For example, phthalate metabolites are 10^+ times greater in urine, but when measuring PCBs and pesticides blood is the preferred matrix. Hair, nails, saliva, sweat, breast milk, feces, and fat tissue biopsies are also used in measuring the concentration of pollutants in the body. Adipose fat tissue testing takes into consideration the long-term bio-accumulation of lipophilic substances and is regarded as a reliable approach in assessing the total body burden, as toxicant levels of many of the chemicals are not often detected in blood or urine testing. The National Health and Nutrition Examination survey includes biomonitoring of >150 chemicals selected for, and based on, the seriousness of known or suspected health effects.

Testing can also assist in designing detoxification protocols for patients. Genova Diagnostics Laboratory located in Asheville, North Carolina offers human biomonitoring assessment of 45 chemicals in their "Toxic Effects CORE Profile – Blood/Urine" test https://www.gdx.net/product/toxic-effects-core-test-urine-blood. Results of the test are lipid adjusted, which reflects a more accurate total body burden of toxicants and allows for those following a cleansing protocol to more closely monitor progress in toxin reduction. Note, however, that this test must be ordered by a physician (and can be expensive.) Customer support representatives at Genova Diagnostics can assist you in locating a physician.

Doctor's Data, located in St. Charles, Illinois also offers testing. Licensed practitioners can order "Toxic and Essential Elements and Environmental Exposure and Detoxification" https://www.doctorsdata.com/environmental/. This test will help clinicians assess the body's capacity for detoxification. Testing is also available that can determine Phase I and Phase II detoxification capacity. The Organix Comprehensive Profile also assesses specific nutrients and B-vitamins that are important for proper mitochondrial functioning of cellular energy. It is available at **https://www.gdx.net/product/organix-com prehensive-profile-metabolic-function-test-urine.**

WEARABLE CHEMICAL MONITORS

The Environmental Defense Fund website has information on a small wearable monitor that detects chemicals that a person comes in contact with. Results of their testing can be found at **https://www.edf. org/health/simple-wristbands-now-detect-chemicalexposure?addl_ info=toxic-chemiclas.** For more information on the MyExposome wristband that tests for chemicals from consumer products, air, and water, visit **http://www.myexposome.com.**

EDUCATIONAL OPPORTUNITIES FOR CEs

Interest in this topic has been expanding at an impressive rate. In the future, interventions to reduce body burdens will become a fundamental part of clinical medicine when biomonitoring becomes a part of every routine annual physical exam. The area of detoxification has primarily attracted interest among practitioners of integrative and complementary medicine practices. Most medical practitioners are untrained in environmental health sciences and courses are not being taught in medical schools, yet practitioners need to be made aware of and be educated in the subject with resources provided in order to educate their patients.

The Centers for Disease Control offers a Pediatric Environmental Health Toolkit Training Module at **https://www.atsdr.cdc.gov/ emes/health_professionals/pediatrics.html.** Also, the University of Arizona's Integrative Medicine program offers the free, 5 credit hour *Environmental Health: An Integrative Approach* available at **https://integrativemedicine.arizona.edu/education/online_courses/ enviro-med.html.**

ADDITIONAL READING MATERIAL

One of the first books to ever document how environmental chemicals affect wildlife was published in 1962, and remains one of the most important science books ever written. Rachel Carson's *Silent Spring* eventually led to a nationwide ban on DDT. How unfortunate that 54 years later we have thousands of new chemicals added to our environment on a daily basis.

At that time there were no books written on detoxification; however, today there are hundreds of books on the market that address the topic. When deciding which books to read first, I would highly recommend beginning with the following, although there are dozens more available:

- *10-Day Detox Diet* – Mark Hyman, MD
- *An A-Z Guide to Food Additives* - Deanna Minich, PhD
- *Clean, Green & Lean – Get Rid of Toxins That Make You Fat* – Walter Crinnion, ND
- *Detox for Life* – Dr. Dan Nuzum
- *Fasting and Eating for Health* – Joel Fuhrman MD and Neal D. Barnard MD
- *Stop the 21st Century Killing You: Toxic Chemicals Have Invaded Our Life* – Paula Baillie-Hamilton, MD, PhD
- *The Detox Box* – Mark Hyman, MD
- *The Detox* Diet – Elson Haas, MD
- *The Toxin Solution* – Dr. Joseph E. Pizzorno
- *Toxic Overload – A Doctor's Plan for Combating the Illnesses Caused by Chemicals in Our Foods* – Paula Baillie-Hamilton, MD, PhD
- *Whole Detox* – Deanna Minich, PhD

CHEMICAL TOXICOLOGICAL EVALUATION DATABASE

The website for the International Programme on Chemical Safety provides toxicological evaluations on over 1,000 chemicals, including a section on pesticide levels in food. It can be accessed at **http://www. inchem.org/pages/jmpr.html.**

CLEAN SCHOOL BUS PROGRAM

The "Clean School Bus" program is designed to reduce children's exposure to emissions, and is available at **https://www.epa.gov/clean diesel/clean-school-bus**

DETERMINING AREAS OF EXPOSURE

When biomonitoring testing is not an option due to cost restrictions, the use of questionnaires can assist in determining exposure. The University of Texas Health Science Center at San Antonio website has an online "Quick Environmental Exposure and Sensitivity Inventory" (QEESI) developed by Dr. Claudia S. Miller. Both physicians and patients can use this questionnaire as a screening instrument. It is available at **http://drclaudiamiller.com/wp-content/ uploads/2012/01/Qeesi.pdf.**

The Centers for Disease Control has published a pdf file on Taking an Exposure History, with CE credit hours available. It can be accessed at **https://www.atsdr.cdc.gov/csem/exphistory/docs/expo sure_history.pdf.** The National Environmental Education Foundation website hosts a "Pediatric Environmental History Form" available at **https://www.neefusa.org/resource/pediatric-environmental-history.**

Dr. Allison Del Bene Davis of the University of Maryland created a "Home Environmental Health and Safety Assessment Tool" available at **https://www.sutterhealth.org/pdf/services/holistic-integra tive-medicine/home-environmental-health-safety-assessment.pdf.**

ENVIRONMENTAL ORGANIZATIONS

Becoming active in any environmental organization or foundation is another way to learn more. Founded in 1998 the Leonardo DiCaprio Foundation is dedicated to working in the areas of climate change, wildland conservation, and protecting biodiversity. Learn more at http://leonardodicaprio.org/. News, videos, blogs and more are available on The Climate Reality Project website including information that provides action steps to get involved in creating a healthier planet - https://www.climaterealityproject.org/.

The Clean Energy Innovation Project website by the Redford Center hosts a plethora of information and videos on endangered waters along with information on a public engagement campaign, available at http://redfordcenter.org/projects/.

The Riverkeeper Organization has been "defending NY's waterways for half a century." The website offers ways to get involved, news and events, and more. It's available at https://www.riverkeeper.org/riverkeeper-mission/.

In 2001 the Oceana Organization was established to focus solely on oceans, and since has protected more than one million square miles of ocean water. Find out more at http://oceana.org/about-oceana/about-us.

Lastly, the Plastic Pollution Coalition website hosts the powerful video "Open Your Eyes" regarding plastic in our waterways. It is available by scrolling down on the following link: http://www.plasticpollutioncoalition.org/.

The World Health Organization's Environmental Pollution webpage provides links to contacts, reports, and activities in regards to the topic: http://www.who.int/phe/en/.

MEDIA RESOURCES

There are also a number of DVDs available documenting the effects that chemicals have on both our bodies and the environment. Check your local library for these and so many others. Search "Environmental Films."

- Earth Report: State of the Planet, 2009
- Libby, Montana, 2007
- Plastic Planet, 2011
- Poisoned Waters, 2009

- The Human Experiment, 2015
- The World According to Monsanto, 2008
- Trashed, 2013

PERSONAL AIR QUALITY MONITORING

Canadian and American air quality can be monitored on the website AirNow available at http://airnow.gov/. To create a better understanding of indoor air quality, also visit the EPA's web page http://www.epa.gov/iaq/pubs/careforyourair.html.

WATER SAFETY DATABASES

The Environmental Working Group's website, the "National Drinking Water Database" is available at http://www.ewg.org/tap-water/. Local drinking water information can be found on the Environmental Protection Agency's website, available at https://www.epa.gov/learn-issues/water-resources#drinking-water. The EPA suggests that drinking water coming from wells should be tested annually or after flooding in the area. Well water can contain high levels of pesticides, volatile organic compounds, and other types of contaminants originating from agricultural or industrial activities. Well water is not regulated by the Environmental Protection Agency.

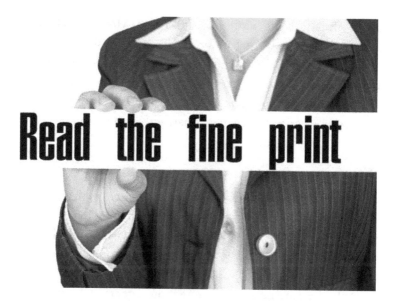

EPILOGUE

While *Your Body's Environmental Chemical Burden* covers several chemicals, it is a mere speck in the scheme of things. The text hasn't touched on the adverse effects of non-ionizing radiation from electromagnetic field exposure originating from wireless and electrical devices found in schools, at work, and in the home. Growing research suggests possible links with brain tumors, childhood leukemia, lymphoma, reproductive dysfunction, chromosomal aberrations, alterations in blood pressure, central nervous system disorders, depression, disruption of sleep patterns, and alterations in brain glucose metabolism.

The health effects of emerging groundwater contaminants and pharmaceutical drugs found in our drinking water include acetaminophen, ibuprofen, primidone, sulfamethoxazole, and DEET are also outside the scope of this book, as is the neurotoxic effect acrylamide demonstrates – a compound we consume by eating low protein, high carbohydrate foods cooked at high temperatures.

Brominated vegetable oils (BVO), utilized as a clouding agent to give a more natural appearance to products, has been used by Pepsico since 1931 and is still found in Fanta, Mountain Dew, and Diet Mountain Dew, yet in Europe BVOs been prohibited for decades with Japan recently discontinuing its use. There are over 4,000 chemical substances in tobacco smoke suspected to be toxic or carcinogenic. Of the 2,500 cleaning products listed by the Environmental Working Group, 53% contain ingredients harmful to the respiratory system.

WHO'S IN CHARGE?

Chemical policies in the U. S. are structured so that the Food and Drug Administration is responsible for cosmetics, food contaminants, medical devices and drug ingredients, yet within the FDA multiple divisions carry out their work in isolation from other departments thereby limiting their concerns to products in their own sector. As an example the Environmental Protection Agency determines whether or not to permit phthalates in a pesticide formula, while the Consumer Products Safety Commission only considers the amount of phthalates that may leach out of a toy as a child chews on it. No single agency is sanctioned to look at the big picture.

THE PARADIGM IS SHIFTING

A paradigm shift in science sometimes occurs painfully slowly due in part to those who won't give up firmly held beliefs, some of which have defined their careers. Paracelsus, a 16th century Swiss German physician, proposed that "the dose makes the poison," however toxicologists today are challenging this outdated assumption because many of the effects of harmful chemicals observed at low doses don't necessarily occur at higher doses, and the opposite has also been observed. Sadly, over the next hundreds of years, humans will be forced to co-exist with the chemicals found in our environment. However, there is hope.

GREEN CHEMISTRY

The director at the Center for Green Chemistry and Green Engineering at Yale, Professor Paul Anastas, contends that chemicals can be designed with an appropriate life cycle and can reduce the use of toxic substances, case in point being the development of green dry-cleaning agents now available. Green building design and construction limits the use of the commonly used toxic chemicals and an International Green Construction Code Book is now available. Eco-Healthy Child Care in California offers a green construction child care endorsement and training program, while Pennsylvania has developed its Early Childhood Education Healthy & Green Initiative. Canada established their Chemicals Management Program in 2006 to protect residents from exposure to harmful chemicals, with important elements of the program including research and biomonitoring of the population. Biological monitoring is and will remain an important tool in assessing personal exposure to chemicals and harmful substances in the environment by determining the overall absorbed dose of humans on an individual basis.

GREEN JOBS MOVEMENT

Outside of research and development, the two largest sectors of the rapidly expanding green jobs movement are in food production and green building. Opportunities to work in water quality control, clean car engineering, biofuel, and recycling are becoming available. There is also a need for solar cell technicians, green design professionals, wave energy producers, and wind energy workers. Each one of these occupations, and more occupations forthcoming in the field, will slowly begin to diminish the use of harmful chemicals in our environment. These fields offer excellent opportunities for young millennials to get involved both occupationally and on a personal health level.

IN CLOSING...

I'd like to express my endless gratitude to the thousands of researchers who share my passion for solving the problem of the body's environmental chemical burden, especially Dr. Stephen Genuis and his group at the University of Alberta in Edmonton Canada, and to all environmental activists and the millennial generation for your time and efforts that will someday (hopefully) correct the mess that's been made of our beautiful planet.

The best course of action one can take is to avoid chemical exposure as much as possible, eat healthy foods as if your life depended upon it, exercise and detoxify daily, revisit the links provided in this book, and become active in helping to spread the word about what we *can* do to change the health of future generations.

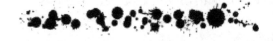

APPENDIX

Agency for Toxic Substances and Disease Registry. Profiles of toxic chemicals. http://www.atsdr.cdc.gov/toxprofiles/index.asp

Agricultural Worker Protection Standards regarding pesticides. https://www.epa.gov/pesticide-worker-safety/agricultural-worker-protection-standard-wps

AirNow. Canadian and American air quality monitoring. http://airnow.gov/

AirOasis. Mobile air sanitizers. https://www.airoasis.com/shop/mobile-purifier/

American Academy of Environmental Medicine. Search by state for a physician. https://www.aaemonline.org/

American College of Occupational and Environmental Medicine. Search by zip code for a physician specializing in environmental health. https://www.acoem.org/DoctorFinderSearch.aspx

Aqua Pure Filters. Activated charcoal filtration and reverse osmosis systems. http://www.aquapurefilters.com/contaminants/150/Pesticides.html

Beyond Pesticides. Organic Christmas trees. http://www.beyondpesticides.org/programs/center-for-community-pesticide-and-alternatives-information/pesticide-free-holidays/christmas

Beyond Pesticides. Triclosan-free products. https://www.beyondpesticides.org/programs/antibacterials/triclosan

Breast Cancer Action. Paraben-free cosmetic companies.
http://www.bcaction.org/our-take-on-breast-cancer/environment/
safe-cosmetics/paraben-free-cosmetics/

Campaign for Safe Cosmetics. Companies voluntarily pledged to
remove chemicals of concern from personal care products.
http://www.safecosmetics.org/get-the-facts/safer-cosmetics-
companies/campaign-safe-cosmetics-compact-signers/

Centers for Disease Control and Prevention. Link to well water testing. http://www.cdc.gov/healthywater/drinking/private/wells/

Centers for Disease Control on Pediatric Environmental Health.
Free continuing education credit course.
https://tceols.cdc.gov/

Centers for Disease Control. "Exposure History Form."
https://www.atsdr.cdc.gov/csem/exphistory/docs/CSEMExposHist-
26-29.pdf

Centers for Disease Control. Working with phthalates.
http://www.cdc.gov/niosh/docs/81-123/pdfs/0236.pdf

ChemSec. Search for producers of hazardous chemicals in Europe:
http://chemsec.org/what-we-do/sin-list

Clean Energy Innovation Project. The Redford Center hosts a
plethora of information and videos on endangered waters along with
information on a public engagement campaign.
http://redfordcenter.org/projects/

Climate Reality Project. Steps to get more involved in creating a
healthier planet. https://www.climaterealityproject.org/

Collaborative on Health and the Environment. 2011 Toxicant and Disease Database. https://www.healthandenvironment.org/our-work/toxicant-and-disease-database/

Collaborative on Health and the Environment. Diseases linked to chemicals, grouped by strength of evidence. https://www.healthandenvironment.org/environmental-health/environmental-risks/

Cornucopia Institute. Organic Eggs Scorecard. http://www.cornucopia.org/organic-egg-scorecard/

Cornucopia Institute. Soy bars and meat alternatives manufactured using hexane solvents. http://www.cornucopia.org/hexane-guides/nvo_hexane_report.pdf

Doctor's Data. "Toxic and Essential Elements and Environmental Exposure and Detoxification." https://www.doctorsdata.com/environmental/

Eco Products. Recyclable dining ware made from sugarcane and bamboo. https://www.ecoproductsstore.com/

Ecology Center of Ann Arbor, Michigan. Healthy gardening tools. http://www.ecocenter.org/healthy-stuff/product-search

Environmental Defense Fund. MyExposome wrist bands to monitor personal chemical exposure. https://www.edf.org/health/simple-wristbands-now-detect-chemical-exposure?addl_info=toxic-chemicals-quiz_trainee5

Environmental Working Group. Skin Deep database of more than 73,000 personal care products. http://www.ewg.org/skindeep/

Environmental Working Group. BPA-lined canned food.
http://www.ewg.org/research/bpa-canned-food

Environmental Working Group. Database on healthy cleaning products. http://www.ewg.org/guides/cleaners

Environmental Working Group. National Drinking Water Database.
http://www.ewg.org/tap-water/

Environmental Working Group. Reducing exposure from BPA.
http://www.ewg.org/research/bpa-in-store-receipts

Etee Products. Alternatives to plastic wraps.
https://www.shopetee.com/

Garden's Alive. Environmentally responsible products for insect and pest control, weed control and other categories.
http://www.gardensalive.com/

Genova Diagnostics Laboratory. "Toxic Effects CORE Profile – Blood/Urine" test.
https://www.gdx.net/product/toxic-effects-core-test-urine-blood

Genova Diagnostics Laboratory. "Organix Comprehensive Profile."
https://www.gdx.net/product/organix-comprehensive-profile-metabolic-function-test-urine

German Human Biomonitoring Commission. Biomonitoring values for more than 130 chemical constituents.
http://www.umweltbundesamt.de/en/topics/chemicals

Healthy Building Network. Building materials and products
http://healthybuilding.net/content/pharos-v3

If You Care. Unbleached paper snack and sandwich.

https://www.ifyoucare.com/

International Programme on Chemical Safety. Toxicological evaluations on over 1,000 chemicals, including a section on pesticide levels in food. http://www.inchem.org/pages/jmpr.html

Lawrence Berkeley National Laboratory. Explanation of air cleaners. https://iaqscience.lbl.gov/air-summary

Leonardo DiCaprio Foundation. Dedicated to working in the areas of climate change, wildland conservation, and protecting biodiversity since 1998. http://leonardodicaprio.org/

Material Safety Data Sheet. Profiles of chemicals. http://www.msds.com/

Medications containing methylparaben. https://www.drugs.com/inactive/methylparaben-290.html

Mighty Nest. Toys free of BPA, phthalates, PVC, formaldehyde, and lead. http://mightynest.com/learn/make-your-nest-mighty/for-your-kids/choosing-safer-toys

National Aeronautics and Space Administration's (NASA) Clean Air Study. https://ntrs.nasa.gov/archive/nasa/casi.ntrs.nasa.gov/19930073077.pdf

National Association for Holistic Aromatherapy. Quality Essential Oils. https://www.naha.org/assets/uploads/The_Quality_of_Essential_Oils_Journal.pdf

National Environmental Education Foundation, "Pediatric Environmental History Form." https://www.neefusa.org/resource/pediatric-environmental-history

National Institutes of Health, National Center for Complementary and Integrative Health. Herb and supplement information. https://nccih.nih.gov/health/atoz.htm

National Sanitation Foundation (NSF International) drinking water filters certified to reduce levels of certain contaminants. http://info.nsf.org/Certified/DWTU/Listings.asp?Trade Name=&Standard=053&ProductType=&PlantState=&Plant Country=&PlantRegion=&submit3=SEARCH&hdModlStd= ModlStd

National Sanitation Foundation (NSF International). Nutritional supplement safety information. http://www.nsf.org/services/by-industry/dietary-supplements/

National Sanitation Foundation (NSF International). Supplement companies in compliance with Good Manufacturing Processes. http://info.nsf.org/Certified/GMP/

Natural Medicines Comprehensive Database. Natural product and drug interaction, nutrient depletion caused by a medication, natural product's effectiveness, and more. http://naturaldatabase.therapeuticresearch.com/home.aspx? cs=&s=ND

New Jersey Department of Health and Senior Services. Hazardous Substance Fact Sheet on Phthalates. http://nj.gov/health/eoh/rtkweb/documents/fs/0765.pdf

Occupational Health and Safety Information on BPA. http://www.bisphenol-a.org/human/occsafety.html

Oceana Organization. Since 2001 has protected more than one million square miles of ocean water. http://oceana.org/about-oceana/about-us

Oregon State University's National Pesticide Information Center. http://npic.orst.edu/envir/testing.html

Penn State University. Information on medicinal plants. http://extension.psu.edu/plants/gardening/herbs

Pesticide Action Network of North America (PANNA). Pesticide Information Database - search by chemical or product name. http://www.pesticideinfo.org/

Plastic Pollution Coalition. Powerful video "Open Your Eyes" regarding plastic in our waterways. It is available by scrolling down on the following link http://www.plasticpollutioncoalition.org/

Professional Artist website. "Ventilating Your Studio" by Louise Buyo. https://professionalartistmag.com/ventilating-your-studio/

Purdue University. Information on medicinal plants. https://hort.purdue.edu/newcrop/Indices/index_ab.html

Rails to Trails Conservancy. https://www.railstotrails.org/

Riverkeeper Organization. Has been "defending NY's waterways for half a century, and hosts information on ways to get involved. http://www.riverkeeper.org/

Rodale's Organic Life. Produce wash recipes. https://www.rodalesorganiclife.com/food/veggie-wash

Santa Cruz Biotechnology datasheet. Occupational exposure to triclosan. http://datasheets.scbt.com/sc-220326.pdf

Seventh Generation. Information on toxic gardening tools. https://www.seventhgeneration.com/blog/toxic-gardening-tools-are-growing-problem

Sloan Kettering Cancer Center. Herbal medicine information. https://www.mskcc.org/cancer-care/diagnosis-treatment/symptom-management/integrative-medicine/herbs/search

Sweetwater Home Water Purification Systems. For well water, kitchen water, reverse osmosis, and a whole house water filtration system. http://cleanairpurewater.com/

Thomas. Chemical supplier or manufacturer database to locate one near your home. Enter zip code in search bar. https://www.thomasnet.com/

United States Department of Agriculture. National directory to Farmer's Markets. https://www.ams.usda.gov/local-food-directories/farmersmarkets

United States Department of Health and Human Services, in cooperation with the National Institutes of Health and the National Cancer Institute. Smoking cessation programs. https://smokefree.gov/

United States Department of Labor, Occupational Safety and Health Administration. Worker's rights and employer responsibilities regarding ventilation at work. https://www.osha.gov/SLTC/ventilation/

United States Department of Labor, Occupational Safety and Health Administration. OSHA enforcement protocols when working with chemicals. https://www.osha.gov/dep/index.html

United States Department of Labor, Occupational Safety and Health Administration. Chemical hazard in nail salons. https://www.osha.gov/SLTC/nailsalons/chemicalhazards.html

United States Department of Labor's Safety and Health Topics. Working with styrene. https://www.osha.gov/SLTC/styrene/

United States Environmental Protection Agency, National Priorities List (NPL) Superfund Sites. https://www.epa.gov/superfund/national-priorities-list-npl-sites-state

United States Environmental Protection Agency. Advisories and Technical Resources for Fish and Shellfish Consumption. https://www.epa.gov/fish-tech

United States Environmental Protection Agency. Agricultural Worker Protection Standards regarding pesticides. https://www.epa.gov/pesticide-worker-safety/agricultural-worker-protection-standard-wps

United States Environmental Protection Agency. Clean School Bus. https://www.epa.gov/cleandiesel/clean-school-bus

United States Environmental Protection Agency. Great Lakes Contaminated Sediments Program. https://www.epa.gov/greatlakes/contaminated-sediment-great-lakes

United States Environmental Protection Agency. Indoor air quality. http://www.epa.gov/iaq/pubs/careforyourair.html

United States Environmental Protection Agency. Local drinking water information. https://www.epa.gov/learn-issues/water-resources#drinking-water

United States Environmental Protection Agency. National Listing of Fish Advisories https://www.epa.gov/fish-tech/national-listing-fish-advisories-general-fact-sheet-2011

United States Environmental Protection Agency. PCBs. https://www.epa.gov/pcbs

United States Environmental Protection Agency. ToxCast. Full listing of genotoxic chemicals. https://www.epa.gov/chemical-research/toxicity-forecasting

United State Food and Drug Administration. National Drug Code Directory. https://www.accessdata.fda.gov/scripts/cder/ndc/index.cfm

United States Food and Drug Administration. Recall information on dietary supplements and foods http://www.fda.gov/food/recallsout breaksemergencies/recalls/default.htm

United States National Library of Medicine. ChemIDplus database of toxic chemicals. https://www.nlm.nih.gov/news/newchemid_04.html

United States National Library of Medicine. Lists chemicals found in products in the following categories: arts & crafts, auto products, commercial/institutional, home maintenance, inside the home, landscape/yard, pesticides, and pet care. Searchable by entering chemical name. https://hpd.nlm.nih.gov/cgi-bin/household/list?tbl=TblChemicals&alpha=A

University of Arizona's Integrative Medicine. "Environmental health: An Integrative Approach." Free continuing education credit course. http://integrativemedicine.arizona.edu/education/online_courses/enviro-med.html

University of California Agriculture and Natural Resources. Soil testing. http://ucanr.edu/sites/UrbanAg/Production/Soils/Soil_Contaminants_and_Soil_Testing/

University of Maryland. "Home Environmental Health and Safety Assessment Tool." https://www.sutterhealth.org/pdf/services/holistic-integrative-medicine/home-environmental-health-safety-assessment.pdf

University of Maryland. Alternative medicine information. http://guides.hshsl.umaryland.edu/pharmacy/cam

University of Texas Health Science Center at San Antonio. "Quick Environmental Exposure and Sensitivity Inventory" (QEESI) developed by Dr. Claudia S. Miller. http://drclaudiamiller.com/wp-content/uploads/2012/01/Qeesi.pdf

University of Wisconsin Integrative Medicine. Detoxification to Promote Health: A 7-Day Program. http://www.fammed.wisc.edu/sites/default/files//webfm-uploads/documents/outreach/im/handout_detoxplan.pdf

Water purification systems. General information on water filtration and distillation systems. http://www.reactual.com/home-and-garden/kitchen-products-2/best-countertop-water-filter.html

What's On My Food. Data extracts from the USDA Pesticide Data Program. http://whatsonmyfood.org/

World Centric Organization. Recyclable serving containers made with wheat straw fiber. http://www.worldcentric.org/

World Health Organization (WHO). Links to contacts, reports, and activities in regards to environmental pollution. http://www.who.int/airpollution/en/

World's Healthiest Foods. Lists of foods high in specific nutrients. http://www.whfoods.com/

GLOSSARY

acetylcholinesterase – an enzyme that stops the signal between nerve and muscle cells

ADHD – attention deficit hyperactivity disorder

adipose tissue – loose connective tissue where fat cells have accumulated

androgenic – refers to male hormones

allergens – something that causes an allergic reaction

Alzheimer's disease – deterioration of the brain's nerve cells

antimicrobial – kills or inhibits the growth of microorganisms

aplastic anemia – bone marrow damage resulting in deficiency of blood cells

arteriosclerosis – hardening of the arteries, also called atherosclerosis or coronary heart disease

atopic dermatitis - eczema

atrophy – wasting away

Autism Spectrum Disorder – impairs a child's ability to interact and communicate with others

b-cells – type of white blood cell, also known as B lymphocytes

battery cages – cramped housing used for egg-laying hens

bioaccumulate – concentrates inside the body

bioavailable – the degree to which something can be absorbed in the body

biomass burning – the burning of plants for land clearing

carcinogen – cancer causing

cardiovascular – heart and blood vessels

central nervous system – brain and spinal cord

chloracne – skin lesions caused by chlorinated chemicals

---

chromosomal deviation – a defect in the normal structure or number of a chromosome

cognitive dysfunction – mental health disorder affecting perception, memory, learning, etc.

colostrum – first secretion from the breast after giving birth, prior to milk

COPD – chronic obstructive pulmonary disorder related to the lungs

cord blood – blood from the umbilical cord

cryptorchidism – undescended testicles

demasculinization – a reduction in masculinity

diabetogenic – producing diabetes

dopamine – chemical that causes the transfer of impulses from one nerve fiber to another

dyslipidemia – elevated LDL (the bad) cholesterol and decreased levels of HDL (the good)

e-waste – electronic appliances and products that have been disposed of

EEG (electroencephalogram) alterations – changes in the electrical activity of the brain detected by a machine

endocrine – gland that secretes hormones into the blood

endocrine disruptors – chemicals that interfere with the body's endocrine system

endometriosis – painful uterine disorder

endothelial – thin tissue that lines the inner surface of blood and lymphatic vessels

Epstein Barr – herpes family virus that can cause mononucleosis, chronic fatigue syndrome

estradiol – most dominant natural estrogen in women produced in the ovaries

estrogen – hormone promoting development and maintenance of female sex characteristics

fasting glucose – blood "sugar" level after not eating for 8 – 12 hours (overnight) *feces* – waste matter eliminated during bowel movement

fetus – unborn child from 8 weeks after fertilization to birth

follicle stimulating hormone – (FSH) pituitary hormone promoting formation of sperm or ova (egg)

fungicide – destroys fungus

GABA – chemical messenger that reduces the activity of the nerve cells to which it binds

genotoxic – destruction of the cells' genetic material

glucose homeostasis – the balance of glucagon and insulin to maintain normal blood "sugar"

half-life – time required for the amount of a substance in the body to decrease by half

hemoglobin – protein containing iron in red blood cells that carries oxygen to tissue

hepatic – relating to the liver

hypertension – high blood pressure

hypospadias – when opening of urethra is found on the underside of the penis

hypothalamic-pituitary-thyroid axis – nerve and hormonal system that regulates metabolism

hypothermia – abnormally low body temperature

idiopathic – condition or disease with an unknown cause

immunosuppressive – suppressing the functioning of an individual's immune system

in utero – in the womb before birth

INF-gamma – regulates the immune response by controlling certain infections and conditions

intestinal lymphatic system – regulates tissue fluid balance, nutrient transport, immune protection

irradiation – exposure to radiation

isomer – a compound with different atom arrangements, but has the same molecular weight *lactation* – milk produced by mammary glands in the breast used to feed the young

leptin resistance – failure of leptin (a hormone produced in fat tissue) to signal fullness

leucocythemia – increased numbers of white blood cells in blood

leukemia – cancer of blood-forming tissues in the body

lipophilic – has a strong affinity for fats

Lou Gehrig's disease – also known as ALS (amyotrophic lateral sclerosis) which is a nerve disease affecting the stimulation of impulses for muscle movement

luteal phase – second half of the menstrual cycle beginning after ovulation

luteinizing hormone – (LH) a hormone stimulating ovulation in women, and the production of male hormones in men

lymphocytes – small white blood cell in the lymphatic system

lymphoma – cancer of the lymph nodes

malignancy – a cancerous tumor

mean platelet volume – blood measurement of the average size of platelets (cells involved in clotting)

meconium – dark green substance passed as first bowel movement in newborn

metabolic syndrome – a group of risk factors raising one's risk of diabetes and cardiovascular disease

metastatic processes – when cancer cells spread to other parts of the body

microorganism – microscopic organism, typically a virus, fungus, or bacterium

mitochondria – structure found in our cells responsible for energy production

mutagen – causes genetic mutation

mutation – altering structure of gene that is passed on to future generations

nanometer – one billionth of a meter

nanoparticles – tiny particle between 1 and 100 nanometers

narcosis – unconsciousness or a dazed state caused by chemicals or pharmaceutical drugs

neurodevelopmental disorders – impaired development of brain functioning becoming more apparent as a child grows

neurological impairment – disorder of the brain and spinal cord such as epilepsy, multiple sclerosis, cerebral palsy, etc.

neuropsychiatric – mental illness attributed to diseases of the brain and nervous system

neuropsychological – human behavior relating to the functioning of the brain and mental functioning

neurotoxic – substance that is poisonous to the brain or nervous tissue

non-Hodgkin's lymphoma – malignant tumor originating from blood cells in the lymphatic system

obesogen – chemical that disrupts hormonal processes in the body and promotes weight gain

off-gassing – release of gas given off a manufactured material or object

oncology – the study of tumors

oxidative damage – imbalance in the body in counteracting or detoxifying harmful effects

particulate matter – particles suspended in air, some of which can be hazardous

peripheral arterial disease – narrowing of arteries that reduce blood flow to the limbs

peripheral neuropathy – damage to nerves causing numbness and pain, especially in the feet and hands

persistent organic pollutants – harmful chemicals that resist breakdown and remain in the environment for a long time

pharmaceuticals – medicinal drugs

phlegm – thick substance secreted from the lungs or the nose

picogram – one trillionth of a gram

placenta – organ that transfers nutrients and oxygen from mother to baby during pregnancy *polycystic ovarian syndrome (PCOS)* – imbalance of estrogen and progesterone hormones in women leading to growth of ovarian cysts

porphyria – abnormal production of the iron-containing pigment that forms hemoglobin

ppb – parts per billion

ppm – parts per million

prolactin – pituitary hormone that signals the production of milk after childbirth

psychomotor – muscular activity or movement associated with mental activity or functioning

pulmonary – relating to the lungs

red blood cell counts – how many red blood cells there are in the blood

sarcoma – cancer developing in soft tissue or connective tissue

semen – white secretion from male reproductive organs containing sperm

sex hormone-binding globulin (SHBG) – protein made in the liver that binds to estradiol and testosterone; marker determining hormonal balance

Social Responsiveness Scale – questionnaire that measures autism spectrum disorder severity

somatic complaints – extreme anxiety about and focus on physical symptoms of pain, fatigue

sperm motility – the percentage of sperm moving in a semen sample

sperm volume – the concentration of sperm in a sample of semen

T lymphocytes – white blood cells that regulate the immune system's response

thymus – a lymph organ that produces T lymphocytes for the immune system

thyroid gland – hormone located in the neck that makes hormones to regulate body temperature, metabolism, heart rate, and blood pressure

thyroid stimulating hormone (TSH) – pituitary hormone that stimulates the thyroid gland to produce T3 and T4

thyrotropin releasing hormone (TRH) – stimulates the release of TSH and prolactin from the pituitary

thyroxine (T4) – main thyroid hormone regulating nearly every process in the body

Total Diet Study (TDS) – annual monitoring of contaminants and nutrients in the average diet

Toxic Substances Control Act -

toxicant – a poisonous substance

triglycerides – major form of fat found in blood and stored in the body's fat cells

triiodothyronine (T3) – thyroid hormone similar to T4 but several times more potent

urogenital tract – organs forming and excreting urine and organs involved in reproduction, such as the male urethra

urethra – the tube that transports urine from the body

visceral obesity – excessive fat deposits protruding from abdominal area

volatile – a substance that evaporates easily at normal temperatures

volatilization – to pass off as vapor

xenobiotic – a substance not normally produced in the body and considered foreign

BIBLIOGRAPHY

INTRODUCTION

Devier MH, Mazellier P, Ait-Aissa S, Budzinksi H. New challenges in environmental analytical chemistry: Identification of toxic compounds in complex mixtures. *C. R. Chimie.* 2011;14:766–779.

Falkowska L, Reindl AR, Szumilo E, Kwasniak J, Staniszewska M, Beldowska M, Lewandowska A, Krause I. Mercury and chlorinated pesticides on the highest level of the food web as exemplified by herring from the Southern Baltic and African penguins from the zoo. *Water Air Soil Pollut.* 2013;224:1549-1563.

Genuis SJ, Tymchak MG. Approach to patients with unexplained multimorbidity with sensitivities. *Canadian Family Physician.* 2014;50:533-539.

Genuis SJ. Fielding a current idea: exploring the public health impact of electromagnetic radiation. *Public Health.* 2008;122:113–124.

Genuis SJ. Pandemic of idiopathic multimorbidity. *Canadian Family Physician.* 2014;60:511-515.

Genuis SJ. Review Article - What's out there making us sick? *Journal of Environmental and Public Health.* Volume 2012, Article ID 605137, 10 pages. doi:10.1155/2012/605137

Genuis SJ. Sensitivity-related illness: The escalating pandemic of allergy, food intolerance and chemical sensitivity. *Science of the Total Environment.* 2010;408:6047–6061.

Genuis SJ. To sea or not to sea: Benefits and risks of gestational fish consumption. *Reproductive Toxicology.* 2008;26:81–85.

Genuis SJ. Toxic causes of mental illness are overlooked. *NeuroToxicology.* 2008;29:1147–1149.

Pugh KH, Zarus GM. The burden of environmental disease in the United States. *Journal of Environmental Health.* 2012;74(9):30-35.

Rauch SA, Lanphear BP. Prevention of Disability in Children: Elevating the Role of Environment. *Future Child.* 2012;22(1):193-217. www.futureofchildren.org

Sears ME, Genuis SJ. Environmental determinants of chronic disease and medical approaches: recognition, avoidance, supportive therapy, and detoxification. *Journal of Environmental and Public Health.* Volume 2012, Article ID 356798, 15 pages. Doi: 10.1155/2012/356798.

Stuart M, Lapworth D, Crance E, Hart A. Review of risk from potential emerging contaminants in UK groundwater. *Science of the Total Environment.* 2012;416:1–21.

Toxicological profile for mirex and chlordecone. U. S. Department of Health and Human Services. Public Health Service Agency for Toxic Substances and Disease Registry. August 1995. http://www.atsdr.cdc.gov/ToxProfiles/tp66.pdf .

Yu GW, Laseter J, Mylander C. Persistent organic pollutants in several different fat compartments in humans. *Journal of Environmental and Public Health.* Volume 2011, Article ID 417980, 8 pages. doi:10.1155/2011/417980

CHAPTER 1 – TOXIC GASES: VOLATILE ORGANIC COMPOUNDS (VOCs)

Amodio A, Dambruoso PR, deGennaro G, deGennaro L, Loiotile AD, Marzocca A, Stasi F, Trizio L, Tutino M. Indoor air quality (IAQ) assessment in a multistory shopping mall by high-spatial-resolution monitoring of volatile organic compounds (VOC). *Environ Sci Pollut Res.* 2014;21:13186–13195.

Delgado-Saborit JM, Aquilina NJ, Meddings C, Baker S, Harrison RM. Relationship of personal exposure to volatile organic compounds to home, work and fixed site outdoor concentrations. *Science of the Total Environment.* 2011;409:478–488.

Elango N, Kasi V, Vembhu B, Poornima JG. Chronic exposure to emissions from photocopiers in copy shops causes oxidative stress and systematic inflammation among photocopier operators in India. *Environmental Health.* 2013;12:78-90.

Estevan C, Ferri F, Sogorb MA, Vilanova E. Characterization and evolution of exposure to volatile organic compounds in the Spanish shoemaking industry over a 5-year period. *Journal of Occupational and Environmental Hygiene.* 2012;9:653–662.

Fuente A, McPherson B, Hickson L. Auditory dysfunction associated with solvent exposure. *BMC Public Health.* 2013;13:39-51.

Geiss O, Barrero-Moreno J, Kotzias D. Measurements of volatile organic compounds in car showrooms in the province of Varese (Northern Italy). *Indoor Air.* 2011;21:45–52.

Ghanem A, Maalouly J, Saad RA, Salameh D, Saliba CO. Safety of Lebanese bottled waters: VOCs analysis and migration studies. *American Journal of Analytical Chemistry.* 2013;4:176-189.

McCready D. A comparison of screening and refined exposure models for evaluating toluene air emissions from a washing machine. *Human and Ecological Risk Assessment.* 2013;19:972–988.

Mohammadi S, Golabadi M, Labbafinejad Y, Pishgahhadian F, Attarchi M. Effects of exposure to mixed organic solvents on blood pressure in non-smoking women working in a pharmaceutical company. *Arh Hig Rada Toksikol.* 2012;63:161-169.

Proctor SP, Heaton KJ, Smith KW, Rodrigues ER, Widing DE, Herrick R, Vasterling JJ, McClean MD. The occupational JP8 exposure neuroepidemiology study (OJENES): repeated workday exposure and central nervous system functioning among US air force personnel. *NeuroToxicology.* 2011;32:799-808.

Sarigiannis DA, Karakitsios SP, Gotti A, Liakos IL, Katsoyiannis. Exposure to major volatile organic compounds and carbonyls in European indoor environments and associated health risk. *Environment International.* 2011;37:743–765.

Sprouse A, Curtis L, Bartlik B. Organic solvent-induced bipolar disorder: a case report. *Adv Mind Body Med.* 2013;27(3):19-23.

Steinemann AC, Gallagher LG, Davis AL, MacGregor IC. Chemical emissions from residential dryer vents during use of fragranced laundry products. *Air Qual Atmos Health.* 2013;6:151–156.

Su FC, Mukherjee B, Batterman S. Trends of VOC exposures among a nationally representative sample: analysis of the NHANES 1988 through 2004 data sets. *Atmospheric Environment.* 2011;45:4858-4867.

Tang T, Gminski R, Kunz M, Modest C, Armbruster B, Mersch-Sundermann V. Investigations on cytotoxic and genotoxic effects of laser printer emissions in human epithelial A549 lung cells using an air/liquid exposure system. *Environmental and Molecular Mutagenesis.* 2012;53:125-135.

Volatile Solvents Guide. Metametrix Clinical Laboratory. Duluth, GA. 2010

BENZENE

Addendum to SUM/140, February 2006 Recommendation from the scientific committee on occupational exposure limits for benzene. SCOEL/SUM/140. European Commission.

American Cancer Society website. 2015. Benzene. Available at: http://www.cancer.org/cancer/cancercauses/othercarcinogens/intheworkplace/benzene. Accessed March 19, 2015.

Barshick SA, Smith SM, Buchanan MV, Guerin MR. Determination of benzene content in food using a novel blender purge and trap GM/MS method. *J of Food Composition and Analysis.* 1995;3:244-257.

Belloc-Santaliestra M, van der Haar R, Molinero-Ruiz E. Occupational exposure assessment of highway toll station workers to vehicle engine exhaust. *Journal of Occupational and Environmental Hygiene.* 2015;12:51–61.

Bogen KT, Sheehan PJ. Dermal versus total uptake of benzene from mineral spirits solvent during parts washing. *Risk Analysis.* 2014;34(7):1336-1359.

Chambers DM, Ocariz JM, McGuirk MF, Blount BC. Impact of cigarette smoking on volatile organic compound (VOC) blood levels in the U.S. Population: NHANES 2003–2004. *Environment International.* 2011;37:1321–1328.

Correa SM, Arbilla G, Marques MRC, Oliveira KMPG. The impact of BTEX emissions from gas stations into the atmosphere. *Atmospheric Pollution Research.* 2012;3:163-169.

Enguita FJ, Leitão AL. Hydroquinone: environmental pollution, toxicity, and microbial answers. *BioMed Research International.* 2013, Article ID 542168, 14 pages http://dx.doi.org/10.1155/2013/542168

Faber J, Brodzik K, Gołda-Kopek A, Łomankiewicz D. Benzene, toluene and xylenes levels in new and used vehicles of the same model. *Journal of Environmental Sciences.* 2013;25(11): 2324–2330.

Fent KW, Eisenberg J, Snawder J, Sammons D, Pleil JD, Stiegel MA, Mueller C, Horn GP, Dalton J. Systemic exposure to PAHs and benzene in firefighters suppressing controlled structure fires. *Ann. Occup. Hyg.* 2014;58(7):830–845.

Huang L, Mo J, Sundell J, Fan Z, Zhang Y. Health risk assessment of inhalation exposure to formaldehyde and benzene in newly remodeled buildings, Beijing. PLoS ONE. 2013;8(11): e79553. doi:10.1371/journal.pone.0079553

Jung KH, Artigas F, Shin JY. Personal, indoor, and outdoor exposure to VOCs in the immediate vicinity of a local airport. *Environ Monit Assess.* 2011;173:555–567.

Kalenge S, Lebouf RF, Hopke PK, Benedict-Dunn RA. Assessment of exposure to outdoor BTEX concentrations on the Saint Regis Mohawk Tribe reservation at Akwesasne New York State. *Air Qual Atmos Health.* 2013;6:181–193.

Kheirbek I, Johnson S, Ross Z, Pezeshki G, Ito K, Eisl H, Matte T. Spatial variability in levels of benzene, formaldehyde, and total benzene, toluene, ethylbenzene and xylenes in New York City: a land-use regression study. *Environmental Health* 2012;11:51. http://www.ehjournal.net/content/11/1/51

Luttrell WE. Benzene. *Journal of Chemical Health & Safety.* July/August 2011:32-33.

Majumdar D, Mukherjeec AK, Mukhopadhayac K, Sen S. Variability of BTEX in residential indoor air of Kolkata metropolitan city. *Indoor Built Environ.* 2012;21(3):374–380.

Mariusz M, Namiesnik J, Zabiegala B. BTEX concentration levels in urban air in the area of the Tri-City agglomeration (Gdansk, Gdynia, Sopot), Poland. *Air Qual Atmos Health.* 2014;7:489–504.

Sahmel J, Devlin K, Burns A, Ferracini T, Ground M, Paustenbach D. An analysis of workplace exposures to benzene over four decades at a petrochemical processing and manufacturing facility (1962–1999). *Journal of Toxicology and Environmental Health.* 2013;Part A:76:723–746.

Santiago F, Alves G, Otero UB, Tabalipa MM, Scherrer LR, Kosyakova N, Ornellas MH, Liehr T. Monitoring of gas station attendants' exposure to benzene, toluene, xylene (BTX) using three-color chromosome painting. *Molecular Cytogenetics.* 2014;7:15. http://www.molecular-cytogenetics.org/content/7/1/15

Scarselli A, Binazzi A, Marzio DD. Occupational exposure levels to benzene in Italy: findings from a national database. *Int Arch Occup Environ Health.* 2011;84:617–625.

Tchepel O, Dias D, Costa C, Santos BF, Teixeira JP. Modeling of human exposure to benzene in urban environments. *Journal of Toxicology and Environmental Health.* 2014;Part A, 77:777–795.

TEACH Chemical Summary. Benzene. U.S. EPA, Toxicity and exposure assessments for children's health. 2009.

ToxGuide for Benzene. U.S. Department of Health and Human Services, Public Health Service, Agency for Toxic Substances and Disease Registry. CAS#71-43-2. October, 2007.

Toxicological review of benzene (non-cancer effects.) Summary Information on the Integrated Risk Information System. EPA/635/R-02/001F

Trevisan P, da Silva JN, da Silva AP, Rosa RFM, Paskulin GA, Thiesen FV, de Oliveira CAV, Zen PRG. Evaluation of genotoxic effects of benzene and its derivatives in workers of gas stations. *Environ Monit Assess.* 2014;186:2195–2204.

US EPA, Office of Air Quality. Locating and estimating air emissions from sources of benzene. EPA-454/R-98-11.

Vinci RM, Jacxsens L, Van Loco J, Matsiko E, Lachat C, de Schaetzen T, Canfyn M, Van Overmeire I, Kolsteren P, De Meulenaer B. Assessment of human exposure to benzene through foods from the Belgian market. *Chemosphere.* 2012;88:1001–1007.

Wallace LA. Major sources of benzene exposure. *Environmental Health Perspectives.* 1989;82:165-169.

Wheeler AJ, Wong SL, Khoury C, Zhu J. Predictors of indoor BTEX concentrations in Canadian residences. *Health Reports.* 2013;24(5):11-17. Statistics Canada, Catalogue no. 82-003-X

Wiwanitkit V. Benzene, cytochrome, carcinogenesis: a topic in preventive toxicology. *Indian J Occup Environ Med.* 2014;18(2): 97–99. doi: **10.4103/0019-5278.146900** PMCID: PMC4280785

World Health Organization. Exposure to Benzene: A major public health concern. 2010. WHO Document Production Services, Geneva, Switzerland

ETHYLBENZENE

Ethylbenzene. Unites States Environmental Protection Agency website. 2013. Available at: **https://www3.epa.gov/airtoxics/hlthef/ethylben.html#ref1.** Accessed March 19, 2015.

Ethylbenzene and Health. Health Canada. 2007. HC Pub 4460.

Ethylbenzene: Production, import/export, use, and disposal. Centers for Disease Control pdf file. Available at: **http://www.atsdr.cdc.gov/toxprofiles/tp110-c5.pdf.** Accessed March 20, 2015.

Luttrell W. Ethylbenzene. *Journal of Chemical Health & Safety.* January/February 2011:41-42.

Su FC, Mukherjee B, Batterman S. Trends of VOC exposures among a nationally representative sample: Analysis of the NHANES 1988 through 2004 data sets. *Atmospheric Environment.* 2011;45:4858-4867.

ToxGuide for Ethylbenzene. Agency for Toxic Substances and Disease Registry. CAS#100-41-4. September 2011.

Toxicological Profile for ethylbenzene. US Dept of Health and Human Services, Public Health Service, Agency for Toxic Substances and Disease Registry, November 2010

STYRENE

13th report on Carcinogens. National Toxicology Program website. 2014. Available at: **http://ntp. niehs.nih.gov/pubhealth/roc/roc13/index.html.** Accessed on March 20, 2015.

Huff J, Infante PF. Styrene exposure and risk of cancer. Mutagenesis. 2011;26(5):583–584 doi:10.1093/mutage/ger033

OPPT Chemical Fact Sheet – Styrene. Environmental Protection Agency CAS No. 100-42-5 available at: http://nepis.epa.gov/Exe/ZyNET.exe/P1004R0Q.TXT?ZyActionD=ZyDocument&Client=EPA&Index=1991+Thru+1994&Docs=&Query=&Time=&EndTime=&SearchMethod=1&TocRestrict=n&Toc=&TocEntry=&QField=&QFieldYear=&QFieldMonth=&QFieldDay=&IntQFieldOp=0&ExtQFieldOp=0&XmlQuery=&File=D%3A\zyfiles\Index%20Data\91thru94\Txt\00000020\P1004R0Q.txt&User=ANONYMOUS&Password=anonymous&SortMethod=h|-&MaximumDocuments=1&FuzzyDegree=0&ImageQuality=r75g8/r75g8/x150y150g16/i425&Display=p|f&DefSeekPage=x&SearchBack=ZyActionL&Back=ZyActionS&BackDesc=Results%20page&MaximumPages=1&ZyEntry=1&SeekPage=x&ZyPURL

Paraskevopoulou D, Achiliasa DS, Paraskevopouloub A. Migration of styrene from plastic packaging based on polystyrene into food stimulants. *Polym Int.* 2012;61:141–148.

Sati PC, Khaliq F, Vaney N, Ahmed T, Tripathi AK, Dev Banerjee B. Pulmonary function and oxidative stress in workers exposed to styrene in plastic factory: Occupational hazards in Styrene-exposed plastic factory workers. *Human and Experimental Toxicology.* 2011;30(11):1743–1750.

Styrene. National Institute of Environmental Health Sciences website. 2014. Available at: http://www.niehs.nih.gov/health/topics/agents/styrene/index.cfm. Accessed March 20, 2015.

Styrene. World Health Organization, Denmark, 2000. Regional office for Europe, Copenhagen, Denmark. Chapter 5.12.

Styrene Hazard Summary. United States Environmental Protection Agency Air Toxics website. 2013. Available at https://www3.epa.gov/airtoxics/hlthef/styrene.html. Accessed March 20, 2015.

Su FC, Mukherjee B, Batterman S. Trends of VOC exposures among a nationally representative sample: Analysis of the NHANES 1988 through 2004 data sets. *Atmospheric Environment.* 2011;45:4858-4867.

Technical Factsheet on Styrene. United States Environmental Protection Agency pdf file. Available at: https://owpubauthor.epa.gov/drink/contaminants/basicinformation/historical/upload/Archived-Technical-Fact-Sheet-on-Styrene.pdf .

Tox Town - Styrene. U.S. National Library of Medicine website. 2014. Available at: https://toxtown.nlm.nih.gov/text_version/chemicals.php?id=87. Accessed on March 20, 2015.

ToxGuide for Styrene. Agency for Toxic Substances and Disease Registry pdf file available at: http://www.atsdr.cdc.gov/toxprofiles/tp53-c5.pdf

Toxicological Profile for Styrene. 2010. U. S. Department of Health and Human Services.

Wongvijitsuka S, Navasumrita P, Vattanasita U, Parnloba V, Ruchirawata M. Low level occupational exposure to styrene: Its effects on DNA damage and DNA repair. *International Journal of Hygiene and Environmental Health.* 2011;214:127–137.

TOLUENE

Hester SD, Johnstone AFM, Boyes WK, Bushnell PH, Shafer TJ. Acute toluene exposure alters expression of genes in the central nervous system associated with synaptic structure and function. *Neurotoxicology and Teratology.* 2011;33:521–529.

Kodavanti PRS, Royland JE, Richards JE, Besas J, MacPhail RC. Toluene effects on oxidative stress in brain regions of young-adult, middle-age, and senescent Brown Norway rats. *Toxicology and Applied Pharmacology.* 2011;256:386–398.

Moroa AM, Bruckera N, Charaoa M, Bulcaoa R, Freitas F, Baierlea M, Nascimentoa S, Valentinic J, Cassinid C, Salvador M, Lindene R, Thiesenf F, Buffonb A, Morescot R, Carcia SC.

Evaluation of genotoxicity and oxidative damage in painters exposed to low levels of toluene. *Mutation Research.* 2012;746:42-48.

Saito A, Tanaka H, Usuda H, Shibata T, Higashi S, Yamashita H, Inagaki N, Nagai H. Characterization of skin inflammation induced by repeated exposure of toluene, xylene, and formaldehyde in mice. *Environmental Toxicology* DOI 10.1002/tox

Shih HT, Yu CL, Wu MT, Liu CS, Tsai CH, Hung DZ, Wu CS, Kuo HW. Subclinical abnormalities in workers with continuous low-level toluene exposure. *Toxicology and Industrial Health.* 2011;27(8):691–699.

The BTX Chain: Benzene, Toluene, Xylene. Chapter 4. The United States Department of Energy. Office of Energy Efficiency and Renewable Energy.

Toluene in Indoor Air. Health Canada website. 2015 Available at: http://www.hc-sc.gc.ca/ewh-semt/pubs/air/toluene/fact-info-eng.php. Accessed March 24, 2015.

Toluene, Chapter 5.14. World Health Organization, Regional Office for Europe, Copenhagen, Denmark. 2000.

Toluene, Hazard Summary. United States Environmental Protection Agency website. 2013. Available at: https://www3.epa.gov/airtoxics/hlthef/toluene.html. Accessed March 24, 2015.

Toluene, Public Health Statement. Agency for Toxic Substances and Disease Registry. 2001.

Toxicological Profile for Toluene. Agency for Toxic Substances and Disease Registry website. 2015. Available at: http://www.atsdr.cdc.gov/toxprofiles/tp.asp?id=161&tid=29. Accessed March 24, 2015.

Walser T, Juraske R, Demou E, Hellweg S. Indoor exposure to toluene from printed matter matters: complementary views from life cycle assessment and risk assessment. *Environ. Sci. Technol.* 2014;48:689–697.

Yang M, Kim SH, Kim JC, Shin T, Moon C. Toluene induces depression-like behaviors in adult mice. *Toxicol. Res.* 2010;26(4):315-320.

XYLENE

Beasley M. Xylene. International Programme on Chemical Safety. Available at: http://www.inchem.org/documents/pims/chemical/xylene.htm#PartTitle:1.%20NAME. Accessed March 21, 2015.

Chronic toxicity summary – Xylenes. Office of the Environmental Health Hazard Assessment California, available at: http://oehha.ca.gov/air/chronic_rels/pdf/xylensREL.pdf

Guideline for Xylene. United States Department of Labor, Occupational Safety and Health pdf file available at: http://www.cdc.gov/niosh/docs/81-123/pdfs/0668.pdf

Luttrell WE. Toxic tips: Xylene. *Journal of Chemical Health & Safety.* 2012:34-35.

Mandiracioglu A, Akgur S, Kocabiyik N, Sener U. Evaluation of neuropsychological symptoms and exposure to benzene, toluene and xylene among two different furniture worker groups in Izmir. Toxicology and Industrial Health. 2011;27(9):802–809.

Toxicological Profile for Xylene. The Agency for Toxic Substances and Disease Registry. 2007. Atlanta, GA

Xylenes Mixed Isomers. United States Environmental Protection Agency Air Toxics website. 2013. Available at: https://www3.epa.gov/airtoxics/hlthef/xylenes.html. Accessed March 21, 2015.

HEXANE

2-Methylpentane. Centers for Disease Control and Prevention website. 2014. Available at: http://www.cdc.gov/niosh/ipcsneng/neng1262.html. Accessed on March 25, 2015.

3-Methylpentane. Centers for Disease Control and Prevention website. 2014. Available at:

http://www.cdc.gov/niosh/ipcsneng/neng1263.html. Accessed on March 25, 2015.

Hexane - Hazard Summary. The United States Environmental Protection Agency website. 2013. Available at: https://www3.epa.gov/airtoxics/hlthef/hexane.html. Accessed on March 25, 2015.

Lampe JW. Is equol the key to the efficacy of soy foods? *Am J Clin Nutr.* 2009;89:1664S-1667S.

Potty VH. Solvent extraction in food industry – a consumer hazard? August 2009. Available at: http://vhpotty.blogspot.com/2009/08/solvent-extraction-in-food-industry.html. Accessed March 25, 2015.

Public Health Statement: n-Hexane. The Agency for Toxic Substances and Disease Registry website. 2015. Available at: http://www.atsdr.cdc.gov/PHS/PHS.asp?id=391&tid=68. Accessed March 25, 2015.

Soy protein and chemical solvents in nutrition bars and meat alternatives. The Cornucopia Institute website. 2010. Available at: https://www.organicconsumers.org/sites/default/files/nvo_hexane_report.pdf . Accessed March 25, 2015.

Swanson BG. Hexane extraction in soyfood processing. Soyfoods Association of North America website. Available at: http://www.soyfoods.org/wp-content/uploads/Regulatory%20Expert%20Document-Barry%20Swanson%20revised.pdf. Accessed March 25, 2015

Toxicological Review of n-Hexane. U.S. Environmental Protection Agency. Available at: http://nepis.epa.gov/Exe/ZyNET.exe/2000E79S.TXT?ZyActionD=ZyDocument&Client=EPA&Index=2000+Thru+2005&Docs=&Query=&Time=&EndTime=&SearchMethod=1&TocRestrict=n&Toc=&TocEntry=&QField=&QFieldYear=&QFieldMonth=&QFieldDay=&IntQFieldOp=0&ExtQFieldOp=0&XmlQuery=&File=D%3A\zyfiles\Index%20Data\00thru05\Txt\00000007\2000E79S.txt&User=ANONYMOUS&Password=anonymous&SortMethod=h|-&MaximumDocuments=1&FuzzyDegree=0&ImageQuality=r75g8/r75g8/x150y150g16/i425&Display=p|f&DefSeekPage=x&SearchBack=ZyActionL&Back=ZyActionS&BackDesc=Results%20page&MaximumPages=1&ZyEntry=1&SeekPage=x&ZyPURL. Accessed on March 25, 2015.

CHAPTER 2 – BANNED BUT PERSISTENT PESTICIDES: CHLORINATED PESTICIDES

Adedeji OB, Okocha RO. Overview of pesticide toxicity in fish. *Environmental Biology.* 2012;6(8):2344-2351.

Alavanja MCR, Ross MK, Bonner MR. Increased cancer burden among pesticide applicators and others due to pesticide exposure. *CA Cancer J Clin.* 2013;63:120–142.

Aprea MC. Environmental and biological monitoring in the estimation of absorbed doses of pesticides. *Toxicology Letters.* 2013;210:110– 118.

Bergman A, Heindel JJ, Kasten T, Kidd KA, Jobling S, Neira M, Zoeller T, Becher G, Bjerregaard P, Bornman R, Brandt I, Kortenkamp A, Muir D, Drisse MNB, Ochieng R, Skakkebaek NE, Bylehn AS, Iguchi T, Toppari J, Woodruff TJ. The impact of endocrine disruption: A consensus statement on the state of the science. *Environ Health Perspect.* 2013;121:a104-a106.

Binnington MJ, Quinn CL, McLachlan MS, Wania F. Evaluating the effectiveness of fish consumption advisories: modeling prenatal, postnatal, and childhood exposures to persistent organic pollutants. *Environ Health Perspect.* 2014;122:178-186.

Bonefeld-Jorgensen EC, Ghisari M, Wielsoe M, Bjerregaard-Olesen C, Kjeldsen LS, Long M. Biomonitoring and hormone-disrupting effect biomarkers of persistent organic pollutants in vitro and ex vivo. *Basic & Clinical Pharmacology & Toxicology.* 2014;115:118–128.

Braun JM, Kalkbrenner AE, Just AC, Yolton K, Calafat AM, Sjodin A. Gestational exposure to endocrine-disrupting chemicals and reciprocal social, repetitive, and stereotypic behaviors in 4- and 5-year-old children: the HOME study. *Environmental Health Perspectives.* 2014;122(5):513-521.

Carpenter SK, Mateus-Pinilla NE, Singh K, Lehner A, Satterthwaite-Phillips D, Bluett RD, Rivera NA, Novakofski JE. River otters as biomonitors for organochlorine pesticides, PCBs, and PBDEs in Illinois. *Ecotoxicology and Environmental Safety.* 2014;100:99–104.

Cho MR, Shin JY, Hwang JH, Jacobs DR, Kim SY, Lee DH. Associations of fat mass and lean mass with bone mineral density differ by levels of persistent organic pollutants: National Health and Nutrition Examination Survey 1999–2004. *Chemosphere.* 2011;82:1268–1276.

Clostre F, Letourmy P, Thuries L, Lesueur-Jannoyer M. Effect of home food processing on chlordecone (organochlorine) content in vegetables. *Science of the Total Environment.* 2014;490;1044–1050.

Crinnion WJ. Chlorinated pesticides: Threats to health and importance of detection. *Altern Med Rev.* 2009;14(4):347-359.

Deribe E, Rosseland BO, Borgstrom R, Salbu B, Gebremariam Z, Dadebo E, Norli HR, Eklo OM. Bioaccumulation of persistent organic pollutants (POPs) in fish species from Lake Koka, Ethiopia: The influence of lipid content and trophic position. *Science of the Total Environment.* 2011;410-411:136–145.

Freire C, Lopez-Espinosa MJ, Fernandez M, Molina JMM, Prada R, Olea N. Prenatal exposure to organochlorine pesticides and TSH status in newborns from Southern Spain. *Science of the Total Environment.* 2011;409:3281–3287.

Hernke MT, Podein RJ. Sustainability, health and precautionary perspectives on lawn pesticides, and alternatives. *EcoHealth.* 2011;8:223–232.

Huang T, Guo Q, Tian H, Mao X, Ding Z, Shang G, Li J, Ma J, Gao H. Assessing spatial distribution, sources, and human health risk of organochlorine pesticide residues in the soils of arid and semiarid areas of northwest China. *Environ Sci Pollut Res.* 2014;21:6124–6135.

Kampire E, Kiremire BT, Nyanzi SA, Kishimba M. Organochlorine pesticide in fresh and pasteurized cow's milk from Kampala markets. *Chemosphere.* 2011;84:923–927.

Kanazawa A, Miyasita C, Okada E, Kobayashi S, Washino N, Sasaki S, Yoshioka E, Mizutani F, Chisaki Y, Saijo Y, Kishi R. Blood persistent organochlorine pesticides in pregnant women in relation to physical and environmental variables in The Hokkaido Study on Environment and Children's Health. *Science of the Total Environment.* 2012;426:73–82.

Kim JT, Lee HK. Metabolic syndrome and the environmental pollutants from mitochondrial perspectives. *Rev Endocr Metab Disord.* 2014;5:253–262.

Lee DH, Liind L, Jacobs DR, Salihovic S, van Bavel B, Lind M. Associations of persistent organic pollutants with abdominal obesity in the elderly: The Prospective Investigation of the Vasculature in Uppsala Seniors (PIVUS) study. *Environment International.* 2012;40:170–178.

Letta BD, Attah LE. Residue levels of organochlorine pesticides in cattle meat and organs slaughtered in selected towns in West Shoa Zone, Ethiopia, Journal of Environmental Science and Health, Part B. *Pesticides, Food Contaminants, and Agricultural Wastes.* 2014;48(1):23-32.

Lu C, Toepel K, Irish R, Fenske RA, Barr DB, Bravo R. Organic diets significantly lower children's dietary exposure to organophosphorus pesticides. *Environ Health Perspect.* 2006;114(2):260-263.Luzardo OP, Almeida-Gonzalez M, Henriquez-Hernandez LA, Sumbado M, Alvarez-Leon EE, Boada LD. Polychlorobiphenyls and organochlorine pesticides in conventional and organic brands of milk: Occurrence and dietary intake in the population of the Canary Islands (Spain). *Chemosphere.* 2013;88:307–315.

Min JY, Cho JS, Lee KJ, Park JB, Park SG, Kim JY, Min KB. Potential role for organochlorine pesticides in the prevalence of peripheral arterial diseases in obese persons: Results
from the National Health and Nutrition Examination Survey 1999–2004. *Atherosclerosis.*
2011;218:200– 206.

Mostafalou S, Abdollahi M. Pesticides and human chronic diseases: Evidences, mechanisms, and
perspectives. *Toxicology and Applied Pharmacology.* 2013;268:157–177.

Polanska K, Jurewicz J, Hanke W. Review of current evidence on the impact of pesticides, polychlorinated biphenyls and selected metals on attention deficit/hyperactivity disorder in children. *International Journal of Occupational Medicine and Environmental Health.* 2013;26(1):16-
38.

Raymer JH, Studabaker WB, Gardner M, Talton J, Quandt SA, Chen H, Michael LC, McCombs
M, Arcury TA. Pesticide exposures to migrant farmworkers in eastern NC: Detection of
metabolites in farmworker urine associated with housing violations and camp characteristics.
Am. J. Ind. Med. 2014;57:323–337.

Reid A, Callan A, Stasinska A, Heyworth, Phi DT, Odland JO, Hinwood A. Maternal exposure to organochlorine pesticides in Western Australia. *Science of the Total Environment.*
2013;449:208–213.

Sengupta P, Banerjee R. Environmental toxins: Alarming impacts of pesticides on male fertility.
Human and Experimental Toxicology. 2014;33(10):1017–1039.

Serveev AV, Carpenter DO. Increase in metabolic syndrome-related hospitalizations in relation
to environmental sources of persistent organic pollutants. *Int. J. Environ. Res. Public Health.*
2011;8:762-776.

Shelton JF, Hertz-Picciotto I, Pessah IN. Tipping the balance of autism risk: Potential mechanisms linking pesticides and autism. *Environ Health Perspect.* 2012;120:944-951.

Stoll ML. Green Chemistry meets green business: A match long overdue. *J Bus Ethics.*
2011;99:23–28.

Valvi D, Mendez MA, Garcia-Esteban R, Ballester F, Ibarluzea J, Go F, Grimalt JO, Llop S,
Marina LS, Vizcaino E, Sunyer J, Vrijheid M. Prenatal exposure to persistent organic pollutants and rapid weight gain and overweight in infancy. *Obesity.* 2014;22:488–496.

Ye M, Beach J, Martin JW, Senthilselvan A. Occupational pesticide exposures and respiratory
health. *Int. J. Environ. Res. Public Health.* 2013;10:6442-6471.

DDT/DDE

Ritter R, Scheringer M, Macleod M, Hungerbuhler K. Nonoccupational exposure to DDT in
humans. *Environmental Health Perspectives.* 2011. 119.5:A194. *Health Reference Center Academic.* Web. 7 Jan. 2015.

Arrebola JP, Mutch E, Rivero M, Choque A, Silvestre S, Olea N, Ocana-Riola R, Mercado
LA. Contribution of sociodemographic characteristics, occupation, diet and lifestyle to DDT
and DDE concentrations in serum and adipose tissue from a Bolivian cohort. *Environment
International.* 2012;38:54–61.

Chlorinated Pesticides Guide. Metametrix Clinical Laboratory, 3425 Corporate Way, Duluth,
GA 30096.

Cohn BA. Developmental and environmental origins of breast cancer: DDT as a case study.
Reproductive Toxicology. 2011;31:302–311.

Crinnion WJ. Chlorinated pesticides: threats to health and importance of detection. *Altern Med
Rev.* 2009;14(4):347-259.

DDT (General Fact Sheet). National Pesticide Information Center. December 1999.

DDT Health Hazard Assessment. International Programme on Chemical Safety. February 2009. World Health Organization.

De Jager C, Aneck-Hahn NH, Bornman MS, Parias P, Spano M. DDT exposure levels and semen quality of young men from a malaria area in South Africa. *Malaria Journal.* 2012,11(1):P21-P22.

Delport R, Bornman R, MacIntyre UE, Oosthuizen NM, Becker PJ, Aneck-Hahn NH, de Japer C. Changes in retinol-binding protein concentrations and thyroid homeostasis with nonoccupational exposure to DDT. *Environ Health Perspect.* 2011;119:647-651.

Dhooge W, den Hond E, Koppen G, Bruckers L, Nelen V, van d Mieroop E, Bilau M, Croes K, Baeyens W, Schoeters G, van Larebeke N. Internal exposure to pollutants and sex hormone levels in Flemish male adolescents in a cross-sectional study: associations and dose-response relationships. *J Expo Sci Environ Epidemiol.* 2011;21(1):106-113.

Fisher A, Walker M, Powell P. DDT and DDE: sources of exposure and how to avoid them. University of Nevada, Cooperative Extension, SP-03-16, NAES #52031334.

Gascon M, Vrijheid M, Martinez D, Ballester F, Basterrechea M, Blarduni E, Esplugues A, Vizcaino E, Grimalt JO, Morales E, Sunyer J. Pre-natal exposure to dichlorodiphenyl-dichloroethylene and infant lower respiratory tract infections and wheeze. *Eur Respir J.* 2012;39:1188–1196.

Giannandrea F, Gandini L, Paoli D, Turci R, Figa-Talamanca I. Pesticide exposure and serum organochlorine residuals among testicular cancer patients and healthy controls. *Journal of Environmental Science and Health,* Part B. 2011;46:780–787.

Govarts E, Nieuwenhuijsen M, Schoeters G, Ballester F, Bloemen K, deBoer M, Chevrier C, Eggesbo M, Guxens M, Kramer U, Legler J, Martinez D, Palkovicova L, Patelarou E, Ranft U, Rautio A, Petersen MS, Slama R, Stifum H, Toft G, Trnovec T, Vandentorren S, Weihe P, Kuperus NW, Wilhelm M, Wittsiepe J, Bonde JP. Birth weight and prenatal exposure to polychlorinated biphenyls (PCBs) and dichlorodiphenyldichloroethylene (DDE): A meta-analysis within 12 European birth cohorts. *Environ Health Perspect.* 2012:120:162-170.

Haugena TB, Tefrea T, Malmc G, Jonssond BAG, Rylanderc L, Hagmard L, Biorsvikb C, Henrichsenb T, Saetherb T, Figenschauf Y, Giwercmanc A. Differences in serum levels of CB-153 and p,p_-DDE, and reproductive parameters between men living south and north in Norway. *Reproductive Toxicology.* 2011;32:261– 267.

Hellou J, Lebeuf M, Rudi M. Review on DDT and metabolites in birds and mammals of aquatic ecosystems. *Environ. Rev.* 2013;21:53–69. dx.doi.org/10.1139/er-2012-0054

Ibarluzea J, Alvarez-Pedrerol M, Guxens M, Marina LS, Basterrechea M, Lertxundi A, Etxeandia A, Goni F, Vioque J, Ballester F, Sunyer J. Sociodemographic, reproductive and dietary predictors of organochlorine compounds levels in pregnant women in Spain. *Chemosphere.* 2011;82:114–120.

Ingber SZ, Buser MC, Pohl HR, Abadin HG, Murray HE, Scinicariello F. DDT/DDE and breast cancer: A meta-analysis. *Regulatory Toxicology and Pharmacology.* 2013;67:421–433.

Kirman CR, Aylward LL, Hays SM, Krishnan K, Nong A. Biomonitoring Equivalents for DDT/DDE. *Regulatory Toxicology and Pharmacology.* 2011;60:172–180.

Latif Y, Sherazi STH, Bhanger MI, Nizamani S. Evaluation of Pesticide Residues in Human Blood Samples of Agro Professionals and Non-Agro Professionals. *American Journal of Analytical Chemistry.* 2012;3:587-595.

Lopes B, Arrebola JP, Serafirm A, Company R, Rosa J, Olea N. Polychlorinated biphenyls (PCBs) and p,p0-dichlorodiphenyldichloroethylene (DDE) concentrations in maternal and umbilical cord serum in a human cohort from South Portugal. *Chemosphere.* 2014;114:291–302.

Mahalingaiah S, Missmer ST, Maity A, Williams PL, Meeker JD, Berry K, Ehrlich S, Perry MJ, Cramer DW, Hauser R. Association of hexachlorobenzene (HCB), dichlorodiphenyltrichloroethane (DDT), and dichlorodiphenyldichloroethylene (DDE) with *in vitro* fertilization (IVF) outcomes. *Environ Health Perspect.* 2012;120:316–320.

Mostafalou S, Abdohhahi M. Pesticides and human chronic diseases: Evidences, mechanisms, and perspectives. *Toxicology and Applied Pharmacology.* 2013;268:157–177.

Neel BA, Sargis RM. The paradox of progress: environmental disruption of metabolism and the diabetes epidemic. *Diabetes.* 2011;60:1838-1849.

Organochlorine Pesticides Overview. Centers for Disease Control and Prevention website. 2013. Accessed June 23, 2015. Available at: http://www.cdc.gov/biomonitoring/DDT_BiomonitoringSummary.html.

Pollack AZ, Buck GM, Lynch CD, Kostyniak PJ. Persistent organochlorine exposure and pregnancy loss: A prospective cohort study. *Journal of Environmental Protection.* 2011;2:683-691.

Tang-Peronard JL, Andersen HR, Jensen TK, Heitmann BL. Endocrine-disrupting chemicals and obesity development in humans: A review. *Obesity Reviews.* 2011;12:622–636.

Turnkvist AT, Glynn A, Aune M, Darnerud PO, Ankarberg EH. PCDD/F, PCB, PBDE, HBCD and chlorinated pesticides in a Swedish market basket from 2005 – Levels and dietary intake estimations. *Chemosphere.* 2011;83:193–199.

U. S. Environmental Protection Agency website. 2011. Accessed June 23, 2015. Available at: https://www3.epa.gov/.

Valvi D, Mendez MA, Martinez D, Grimalt JO, Torrent M, Sunyer J, Vrijheid M. Prenatal Concentrations of polychlorinated biphenyls, DDE, and DDT and overweight in children: A prospective birth cohort study. *Environ Health Perspect.*2012;120:451-457.

Vogt R, Bennett D, Cassady D, Frost J, Ritz B, Hertz-Picciotto I. Cancer and non-cancer health effects from food contaminant exposures for children and adults in California: a risk assessment. *Environmental Health.* 2012;11:83-97.

ALDRIN AND DIELDRIN

Aldin and Dieldrin CAS # 309-00-2 and 60-57-1. ToxFAQs. Agency for Toxic Substances and Disease Registry (ATSDR). 2002. Toxicological Profile for Aldrin/Dieldrin. Atlanta, GA: U.S. Department of Health and Human Services, Public Health Service.

Chlorinated Pesticides Guide. Metametrix Clinical Laboratory, 3425 Corporate Way, Duluth, GA 30096.

Crinnion WJ. Chlorinated pesticides: threats to health and importance of detection. *Altern Med Rev.* 2009;14(4):347-359.

Health Effects Support Document for Aldrin/Dieldrin. U.S. Environmental Protection Agency Office of Water. Health and Ecological Criteria Division Washington, DC 20460. EPA 822-R-03-001February 2003

Public Health Statement Aldrin and Dieldrin. CAS# 309-00-2 & 60-57-1. Sept 2002. Agency for Toxic Substances and Disease Registry (ATSDR).

Stern AH. Hazard identification of the potential for dieldrin carcinogenicity to humans. *Environmental Research.* 2014;131:188–214.

Yu GW, Laseter J, Mylander C. Persistent organic pollutants in serum and several different fat compartments in humans. *Journal of Environmental and Public Health.* 2011. Article ID 417980, 8 pages. doi:10.1155/2011/417980

HEPTACHLOR

Heptachlor. U.S. Agency for Toxic Substances and Disease Registry. Public Health Statement. Heptachlor 76-44-8. Hazard Summary-Created in April 1992; Revised in January 2000. United States Environmental Protection Agency website. October 2013. Accessed July 8, 2015. Available at: http://www.epa.gov/ttnatw01/hlthef/heptachl.html

Heptachlor and Heptachlor Epoxide in Drinking-water. Background document for development of WHO Guidelines for Drinking-water Quality. WHO/SDE/WSH/03.04/99. World Health Organization 2004.

Luderer U, Kesner JS, Fuller JM, Krieg EF, Meadows JW, Tramma SL, Yang H, Baker D. Effects of gestational and lactational exposure to heptachlor epoxide on age at puberty and reproductive function in men and women. *Environmental Research*. 2013;121:84-94.

R.E.D. FACTS Heptachlor Pesticide Reregistration Eligibility Document. United States Environmental Protection Agency. Prevention, Pesticides and Toxic Substances (7508W). 738-F-92-002, March 1992.

Toxicological Profile for Heptachlor/Heptachlor Epoxide. U. S. Department of Health and Human Services. Public Health Service Agency for Toxic Substances and Disease Registry. April 1993

HEXACHLOROBENZENE

Agency for Toxic Substances and Disease Registry (ATSDR). *Toxicological Profile for Hexachlorobenzene*. Public Health Service, U.S. Department of Health and Human Services, Atlanta, GA. 1996.

Chlorinated Pesticides Guide. Metametrix Clinical Laboratory, 3425 Corporate Way, Duluth, GA 30096.

Crinnion WJ. Chlorinated pesticides: threats to health and importance of detection. *Altern Med Rev*. 2009;14(4):347-359.

Hexachlorobenzene. Hazard Summary-Created in April 1992; Revised in January 2000. 118-74-1. Available at: https://www3.epa.gov/airtoxics/hlthef/hexa-ben.html.

Lama T, Williams PL, Lee MM, Korrick SA, Birnbaum LS, Burns JS, Sergeyey O, Revich B, Altshul LM, Patterson, DG, Turner WE, Hauser R. Prepubertal organochlorine pesticide concentrations and age of pubertal onset among Russian boys. *Environment International*. 1024;73:135–142.

Mrema EJ, Rubino FM, Mandic-Rajcevic S, Sturchio E, Turci R, Osculati A, Brambilla G, Minoia C, Colosio C. Exposure to priority organochlorine contaminants in the Italian general population. Part 1. Eight priority organochlorinated pesticides in blood serum. *Human and Experimental Toxicology*. 2013;32(12):1323–1339.

Park JS, Shin SK, Kim WI, Kim BH. Residual levels and identify possible sources of organochlorine pesticides in Korea atmosphere. *Atmospheric Environment*. 2011;45:7496-7502.

Perello G, Gomez-Catalan J, Castell V, Lobet JM, Domingo JL. Estimation of the daily intake of hexachlorobenzene from food consumption by the population of Catalonia, Spain: Health risks. *Food Control*. 2012;23:198-202.

Song S, Mab J, Tian Q, Tong L, Guo X. Hexachlorobenzene in human milk collected from Beijing, China. *Chemosphere*. 2013;91:145–149.

Toxic Effects Porphyrins Profile Interpretive Guide. Metametrix – ©2007-2008 Metametrix, Inc.

Toxicological Profile for Hexachlorobenzene. Update. September 30, 2013.

Upson K, De Roos AJ, Thompson ML, Sathyanarayana S, Scholes D, Barr DB, Holt VL.

Organochlorine pesticides and risk of endometriosis: findings from a population-based case-control study. *Environ Health Perspect.* 2013;121:1319-1324.

Zhou P, Zhao Y, Li J, Wu G, Zhang L, Liu Q, Fan S, Yang X, Li X, Wu Y. Dietary exposure to persistent organochlorine pesticides in 2007 Chinese total diet study. *Environment International.* 2012;42:152–159.

MIREX

Biomonitoring Summary, Organochlorine Pesticides Overview. Centers for Disease Control and Prevention website. 2013. Accessed July 9, 2013. Available at: http://www.cdc.gov/biomonitoring/Mirex_BiomonitoringSummary.html

Chlorinated Pesticides Guide. Metametrix Clinical Laboratory, 3425 Corporate Way, Duluth, GA 30096.

Crinnion WJ. Chlorinated pesticides: threats to health and importance of detection. *Altern Med Rev.* 2009:14(4):347-359.

Mirex, CAS No. 2385-85-5. Agency for Toxic Substances and Disease Registry (ATSDR). Toxicological profile for mirex and chlordecone. August 1995.

Persistent Organic Pollutants Toolkit. The Canadian International Development Agency website. Accessed July 9, 2015. Available at: http://www-esd.worldbank.org/popstoolkit/POPsToolkit/POPSTOOLKIT_COM/ABOUT/CHEMICAL/MIREX.HTM

Report on Carcinogens, Thirteenth Edition. National Toxicology Program, United States Department of Health and Human Services website. 2015. Accessed July, 2015. Available at: http://ntp.niehs.nih.gov/pubhealth/roc/roc13/index.html

Toxic Substances Portal – Mirex. Agency for Toxic Substances & Disease Registry website. 2015. Accessed July 9, 2015. Available at: http://www.atsdr.cdc.gov/toxprofiles/tp.asp?id=1190&tid=276

CHLORDANE

Crinnion WJ. Chlorinated pesticides: threats to health and importance of detection. *Altern Med Rev.* 2009;14(4):347-359.

Environmental Health – Infrastructure and Surveillance. HealthyPeople.gov website. 2015. Accessed July 9, 2015. Available at: https://www.healthypeople.gov/2020/topics-objectives/topic/environmental-health/objectives

National Biomonitoring Program. Centers for Disease Control and Prevention website. Accessed July 9, 2015. Available at: http://www.cdc.gov/biomonitoring/ChlordaneHeptachlor_BiomonitoringSummary.html

Neta G, Goldman LR, Barr D, Apelberg BJ, Witter FR, Halden RU. Fetal exposure to chlordane and permethrin mixtures in relation to inflammatory cytokines and birth outcomes. *Environmental Science and Technology.* 2011;45:1680-1687.

Oxychlordane. TOXNET, Toxicology Data Network. National Library of Medicine website. 2003. Accessed July, 2015. Available at: http://toxnet.nlm.nih.gov/cgi-bin/sis/search/a?dbs+hsdb:@term+@DOCNO+6771

Toxic Substances Portal – Chlordane. Agency for Toxic Substances & Disease Registry website. 2015. Accessed July 9, 2015. Available at: http://www.atsdr.cdc.gov/ToxProfiles/tp.asp?id=355&tid=62#bookmark06

Toxicological profile for chlordane. U. S. Department of Health and Human Services. Public Health Service. Agency for Toxic Substances and Disease Registry. May 1994

Trabert B, Longnecker MP, Brock JW, Klebanoff MA, McGlynn KA. Maternal pregnancy levels of *trans*-nonachlor and oxychlordane and prevalence of cryptorchidism and hypospadias in boys. *Environmental Health Perspectives.* 2012;120(3):478-482.

ENDOSULFAN

ATSDR. Public Health Statement. Endosulfan. June 2013. Atlanta, GA.

Beauvais SL, Silva MH, Powell S. Human health risk assessment of endosulfan. Part III: Occupational handler exposure and risk. *Regulatory Toxicology and Pharmacology.* 2010;56;28–37.

Beauvais SL, Silva MH, Powell S. Human health risk assessment of endosulfan. Part IV: Occupational reentry and public non-dietary exposure and risk. *Regulatory Toxicology and Pharmacology.* 2010;56:38–50.

Beauvais SL, Silva MH, Powell S. Human health risk assessment of endosulfan. Part III: Occupational handler exposure and risk. *Regulatory Toxicology and Pharmacology.* 2010;56;28–37.

Desalegn B, Takasuga T, Harada KH, Hitomi T, Fujii Y, Yang HR, Wang P, Senevirathna STMLD, Koisumi A. Historical trends in human dietary intakes of endosulfan and toxaphene in China, Korea and Japan. *Chemosphere.* 2011;83:1398–1405.

EPA Action to Terminate Endosulfan. United States Environmental Protection Agency website. 2015. Accessed July 9, 2015. Available at: https://archive.epa.gov/pesticides/reregistration/web/html/endosulfan-cancl-fs.html.

Rau ATK, Coutinho A, Avabratha KS, Rau AR, Warrier RP. Pesticide (Endosulfan) levels in the bone marrow of children with hematological malignancies. *Indian Pediatrics.* 2012;49:113-119.

Silva MH, Beauvais SL. Human health risk assessment of endosulfan: I. Toxicology and hazard identification. *Regulatory Toxicology and Pharmacology.* 2010;56:4-17.

Silva MH, Carr WC. Human health risk assessment of endosulfan: II. Dietary exposure assessment. *Regulatory Toxicology and Pharmacology.* 2010;56:18-27.

United States Prevention, Pesticides EPA 738-R-02-013. Environmental Protection and Toxic Substances Agency (7508C). November 2002

CHAPTER 3 – MOST WIDELY USED PESTICIDES TODAY:
ORGANOPHOSPHATE PESTICIDES

Alcala LQ, Alkon AD, Boyce WT, Lippert S, Davis NV, Bradman A, Barr DB, Eskenazi B. Maternal prenatal and child organophosphate pesticide exposures and children's autonomic function. *NeuroToxicology.* 2011;32:646–655.

Alcala LQ, Bradman A, Smith K, Weerasekera G, Odetokun M, Barr DB, Nishioka M, Castorinal R. Hubbard AE. Nicas M. Hammond K, McKone TE, Eskenazi B. Organophosphorous pesticide breakdown products in house dust and children's urine. *Journal of Exposure Science and Environmental Epidemiology.* 2012;22:559-568.

Atrazine. Volume 73. IARC Monographs.

Atrazine Current Updates. January 2013. United States Environmental Protection Agency website. 2015. Accessed August 11, 2015. Available at: https://archive.epa.gov/pesticides/reregistration/web/html/status.html

Barr DB, Clune AL, Ryan BP. Have regulatory efforts to reduce organophosphorus insecticide exposures been effective? *Environmental Health Perspectives.* 2012;120(4):521-526.

Barr DB, Wong LY, Bravo R, Weerasekera G, Odetokun M, Restrepo P, Kim DG, Fernandez C, Whitehead RD, Perez J, Gallegos M, Williams BL, Needham LL. Urinary concentrations of dialkylphosphate metabolites of organophosphorus pesticides: National Health and Nutrition Examination Survey 1999–2004. *Int. J. Environ. Res. Public Health.* 2011;8:3063-3098.

Beamer PI, Canales RA, Ferguson AC, Leckie JO, Bradman A. Relative pesticide and exposure route contribution to aggregate and cumulative dose in young farmworker children. *Int. J. Environ. Res. Public Health.* 2012;9:73-96.

Biomonitoring California. Dimethylthiophosphate (DMTP). CAS Number 1112-38-5. CA.gov website. 2015. Accessed August 10, 2015. Available at: http://biomonitoring.ca.gov/chemicals/dimethylthiophosphate-dmtp

Biomonitoring Summary. Organophosphorus insecticides: Dialkyl phosphate metabolites. Centers for Disease Control and Prevention website. 2013. Accessed August 10, 2015. Available at: http://www.cdc.gov/biomonitoring/OP-DPM_BiomonitoringSummary.html

Bottoni P, Grenni P, Lucentini L, Caracciolo AB. Terbuthylazine and other triazines in Italian water resources. *Microchemical Journal.* 2013;107:136–142.

Bouchard MF, Chevrier J, Harley KG, Kogut K, Vedar M, Calderon N, Trujillo C, Johnson C, Bradman A, Barr DB, Eskenazi B. Prenatal exposure to organophosphate pesticides and IQ in 7-year-old children. *Environ Health Perspect.* 2011;119:1189–1195.

Bradman A, Castorina R, Barr DB, Chevrier J, Harnly ME, Eisen EA, McKone TE, Harley K, Holland N, Eskenazi B. Determinants of organophosphorus pesticide urinary metabolite levels in young children living in an agricultural community. *Int. J. Environ. Res. Public Health.* 2011;8:1061-1083.

Chevrier C, Limon G, Monfort C, Rouget F, Garlantezec R, Petit C, Durand G, Cordier S. Urinary biomarkers of prenatal atrazine exposure and adverse birth outcomes in the PELAGIE birth cohort. *Environ Health Perspect.* 2011;119:1034-1041.

Cragin LA, Kesner JS, Bachand AM, Barr DB, Meadows JW, Krieg EF, Reif JS. Menstrual cycle characteristics and reproductive hormone levels in women exposed to atrazine in drinking water. *Environmental Research.* 2011;111:1293-1301.

Decision Documents for Atrazine. 2003. United States Environmental Protection Agency, Washington, DC. Office of Prevention, Pesticides and Toxic Substances.

Esquivel-Senties MS, Esquivel-Senties LV, Vega L. Organophosphorous pesticides metabolite reduces human T CD8 homeostasis and proliferation by inducing cellular death. *J Environment Analytic Toxicol.* 2012;8(4). doi:10.4172/2161-0525.S4-004.

General Information. Atrazine CAS# 1912-24-9. September 2003. Department of Health and Human Services, Public Health Service Agency for Toxic Substances and Disease Registry.

Gution ToxFAQs, CAS 86-50-0. Department of Health and Human Services, Public Health Service Agency for Toxic Substances and Disease Registry.

Li Y, Sun Y, Yang J, Wu Y, Yu J, Li B. The long-term effects of the herbicide atrazine on the dopaminergic system following exposure during pubertal development. *Mutation Research* 2014;763:23-29.

McKelvey W, Jacobson JB, Kass D, Barr DB, Davis M, Calafat A, Aldous KM. Population-based biomonitoring of exposure to organophosphate and pyrethroid pesticides in New York City. *Environ Health Perspect.* 2013;121:1349-1356.

National Health and Nutrition Examination Survey 2007 - 2008 Data Documentation, Codebook, and Frequencies Organophosphate Insecticides - Diakyl Phosphate Metabolites – Urine. Data File: OPD_E.xpt. May, 2012. Available at: http://wwwn.cdc.gov/nchs/nhanes/2007-2008/OPD_E.htm

Organophosphate Pesticides. National Report on Human Exposure to Environmental Chemicals. Centers for Disease Control and Prevention, Atlanta, Georgia. Mar01. Mindfully.org website. Accessed August 10, 2015. http://www.mindfully.org/Pesticide/Organophosphate-Pesticides-CDCMar01.htm.

Organophosphates Profile Guide. Metametrix Clinical Laboratory. Duluth, GA.

Organophosphates. Pesticide Action Network of North America website. Accessed August 10, 2015. http://www.panna.org/resources/organophosphates.

Organophosphorus Cumulative Risk Assessment – 2006 Update. August 2006, USEPA. Technical Executive Summary.

Peighambarzadeh SZ, Safi S, Shahtaheri SJ, Javanbakht M, Forushani AR. Presence of atrazine in the biological samples of cattle and its consequence adversity in human health. *Iranian J Publ Health*. 2011;40(4)112-121.

Perry MJ, Venners SA, Chen X, Lui X, Tang G, Xing H, Barr DB, Xue X. Organophosphorous pesticide exposures and sperm quality. *Reproductive Toxicology*. 2011;31:75–79.

Public health statement Atrazine CAS#1912-24-9. Department of Health and Human Services, Public Health Service Agency for Toxic Substances and Disease Registry.

Public health statement Chlorpyrifos CAS#2921-88-2, August 1998. Department of Health and Human Services, Public Health Service Agency for Toxic Substances and Disease Registry.

Public health statement Diazinon CAS# 333-41-5, September 2008. Department of Health and Human Services, Public Health Service Agency for Toxic Substances and Disease Registry.

Public Health Statement Disulfoton. CAS#:298-04-4. August 1995. Department of Health and Human Services, Public Health Service Agency for Toxic Substances and Disease Registry.

Public Health Statement Ethion CAS# 563-12-2. September 2000. Department of Health and Human Services, Public Health Service Agency for Toxic Substances and Disease Registry.

Public Health Statement Malathion, CAS# 121-75-5 September 2003. Department of Health and Human Services, Public Health Service Agency for Toxic Substances and Disease Registry.

Public health statement Methyl parathion CAS# 298-00-0, September 2001. Department of Health and Human Services, Public Health Service Agency for Toxic Substances and Disease Registry.

Rinsky JL, Hopenhayn C, Golla V, Browning S, Bush HM. Atrazine exposure in public drinking water and preterm birth. *Public Health Reports*. 2012;127:72-81.

Rygwelski KR, Zhang X, Kreis RG. Model forecasts of atrazine in Lake Michigan in response to various sensitivity and potential management scenarios. *Journal of Great Lakes Research*. 2012;38:1-10.

Saunders M, Magnanti BL, Carreira SC, Yang A, Alamo-Hernandez U, Riojas-Rodriguez H, Calmandrei G, Koppe JG, von Krauss MK, Keune H, Bartonova A. Chlorpyrifos and neurodevelopmental effects: a literature review and expert elicitation on research and policy. *Environmental Health*. 2012;11(1):55-66.

Surface water and drinking water in the United States. Natural Resources Defense Council. April 2010. Still Poisoning the Well.

ToxFAQ. Dichlorvos CAS # 62-73-7. September 1997. Department of Health and Human Services, Public Health Service Agency for Toxic Substances and Disease Registry.

Trouble on the farm: Growing up with pesticides in agricultural communities. The Natural Resource Defense Council website. Accessed August 10, 2015. Available at: https://www.nrdc.org/stories/24-d-most-dangerous-pesticide-youve-never-heard

Ueyama J, Saito I, Kondo T, Taki T, Kimata A, Saito S, Ito Y, Murata K, Iwata T, Gotoh M, Shibata E, Wakusawa S, Kamijima M. Urinary concentrations of organophosphorus insecticide metabolites in Japanese workers. *Chemosphere*. 2012;87:1403–1409.

Ueyama J, Saito I, Takaishi A, Nomura H, Inoue M, Osaka A, Sugiura Y, Hayashi Y, Wakusawa S, Ogi H, Inuzuka K, Kamijima M, Kondo T. A revised method for determination of dialkylphosphate levels in human urine by solid-phase extraction and liquid chromatography with tandem mass spectrometry: application to human urine samples from Japanese children. *Environ Health Prev Med.* 2014;19:405–413.

Wang P, Tian Y, Wang XJ, Gao Y, Shi R, Wang GQ, Hu GH, Shen XM. Organophosphate pesticide exposure and perinatal outcomes in Shanghai, China. *Environment International.* 2012;42:100–104.

Wu M, Quirindongo M, Sass J, Wetzler A. Atrazine continues to contaminate surface water and drinking water in the United States. National Resources Defense Council. 2010.

Yolton K, Xu Y, Sucharew H, Succop P, Altaye M, Popelar A, Montesano MA, Calafat AM, Khoury JC. Impact of low-level gestational exposure to organophosphate pesticides on neuro-behavior in early infancy: a prospective study. *Environmental Health.* 2013;12:79-89.

Chapter 4 – Chemicals Used in Plastics Manufacturing: Polychlorinated Biphenyls (PCBs)

Asante KA, Adu-Kumi S, Nakahiro K, Takahashi S, Isobe T, Sudaryanto A, Devanathan G, Clarke E, Ansa-Asare OD, Dapaah-siakwan S, Tanabe S. Human exposure to PCBs, PBDEs and HBCDs in Ghana: Temporal variation, sources of exposure and estimation of daily intakes by infants. *Environment International.* 2011;37:921–928.

Aylward LL, Collins JJ, Bodner KM, Wilken M, Bodnar CM. "Intrinsic" elimination rate and dietary intake estimates for selected indicator PCBs: Toxicokinetic modeling using serial sampling data in US subjects, 2005–2010. *Chemosphere.* 2014;110:48–52.

Boix J, Cauli O. Alteration of serotonin system by polychlorinated biphenyls exposure. *Neurochemistry International.* 2012;60:809–816.

Brunelli L, Lansola ML, Felipo V, Campagna R, Airold L, De Paola M, Fanell R, Marian A, Mazzolett M, Pastorelli R. Insight into the neuroproteomics effects of the food-contaminant non-dioxin like polychlorinated biphenyls. *Journal of Proteomics.* 2012;75:2417-2430.

Caudle WM, Guillot TS, Lazo CR, Miller GW. Industrial toxicants and Parkinson's disease. *NeuroToxicology.* 2012;33:178–188.

Cho MR, Shin JY, Hwang JH, Jacobs DR, Kim SY, Lee DH. Associations of fat mass and lean mass with bone mineral density differ by levels of persistent organic pollutants: National Health and Nutrition Examination Survey 1999–2004. *Chemosphere.* 2011;82:1268–1276.

Cimenci O, Vandevijvere S, Boscinny S, Van Den Bergh MA, Hanot V, Vinkx C, Bolle F, Van Loco J. Dietary exposure of the Belgian adult population to non-dioxin-like PCBs. *Food and Chemical Toxicology.* 2013;59:670–679.

Cohna BA, Cirillo PM, Scholtza RI, Ferrarab A, Park JS, Schwing PJ. Polychlorinated biphenyl (PCB) exposure in mothers and time to pregnancy in daughters. *Reproductive Toxicology.* 2011;31:290–296.

Cok I, Mazmanci B, Mazmanci MA, Turgut C, Henkelmann B, Schramm KW. Analysis of human milk to assess exposure to PAHs, Pcbs and organochlorine pesticides in the vicinity Mediterranean city Mersin, Turkey. *Environment International.* 2012;40:63–69.

Committees on Toxicity, Mutagenicity, Carcinogenicity of Chemicals in Food, Consumer Products and the Environment. Annual Report 2007. United Kingdom. Task 4-Human Exposure, Annex 2. Contribution of PCBs to Total TEQ Exposure. AEA Technology.

Crinnion WJ. Polychlorinated biphenyls: Persistent pollutants with immunological, neurological, and endocrinological consequences. *Alternative Medicine Review.* 2011;16(1):5-19.

Dickerson SM, Cunningham SL, Patisaul HB, Woller MJ, Gore AC. Endocrine disruption of brain sexual differentiation by developmental PCB exposure. *Endocrinology.* 2011;152(2):581–594.

Dioxins and their effects on human health. The World Health Organization website. 2015. Accessed July 24, 2015. Available at: http://www.who.int/mediacentre/factsheets/fs225/en/

Elabbas LE, Finnila MA, Herlin M, Stern N, Trossvik C, Bowers WJ, Nakai J, Tukkanen J, Heimeier RA, Akesson A, Hakansson H. Perinatal exposure to environmental contaminants detected in Canadian Arctic human populations changes bone geometry and biomechanical properties in rat offspring. *Journal of Toxicology and Environmental Health*, Part A: Current Issues. 2011;74(19):1304-1318.

Eske K, Newsome B, Han SG, Murphy M, Bhattacharyya D, Hennig B. PCB 77 dechlorination products modulate pro-inflammatory events in vascular endothelial cells. *Environ Sci Pollut Res*. 2014;21:6354–6364.

Exposure to dioxins and dioxin-like substances: A major public health concern. World Health Organization website. 2010. Accessed July 24, 2015. Available at: http://www.who.int/ipcs/features/dioxins.pdf

Ferguson KK, Hauser R, Altshul L, Meeker JD. Serum concentrations of p, p_-DDE, HCB, PCBs and reproductive hormones among men of reproductive age. *Reproductive Toxicology*. 2012;34:429–435.

Ferguson KT, Cassells RC, MacAllister JW, Evans GW. The physical environment and child development: An international review, *International Journal of Psychology*. 2013;48(4):437-468.

Ferrante MC, Amer P, Santor A, Monnol A, Simeol R, Di Guida F, Raso GM, Meli R. Poly-chlorinated biphenyls (PCB 101, PCB 153 and PCB 180) alter leptin signaling and lipid metabolism in differentiated 3T3-L1 adipocytes. *Toxicology and Applied Pharmacology*. 2014;279:401–408.

Ferrante MC, Raso GM, Espositoc E, Biancod G, Iaconob A, Clausia MT, Amerob P, Santorob A, Simeolib R, Autored G, Meli R. Effects of non-dioxin-like polychlorinated biphenyl con-geners (PCB 101, PCB 153 and PCB 180) alone or mixed on J774A.1 macrophage cell line: modification of apoptotic pathway. *Toxicology Letters*. 2011;202:61–68.

Fromberg A, Granby K, Hojgard A, Fagt S, Larsen JC. Estimation of dietary intake of PCB and organochlorine pesticides for children and adults. *Food Chemistry*. 2011;125:1179–1187.

Gascon M, Verner MA, Guxens M, Grimalt JO, Forns J, Ibarluzea J, Lertxundi N, Ballester F, Llop S, Haddad S, Sunyer J, Vrijheid M. Evaluating the neurotoxic effects of lactational exposure to persistent organic pollutants (POPs) in Spanish children. *NeuroToxicology*. 2013;34:9–15.

Ghosh S, Zang S, Mitra PS, Ghimboyschi S, Hoffman EP, Dutta SK. Global gene expression and ingenuity biological functions analysis on PCBs 153 and 138 induced human PBMC in vitro reveals differential mode(s) of action in developing toxicities. *Environment International*. 2011;37:838–857.

Gioia R, Akindele AJ, Adebusoye SA, Asante KA, Tanabe S, Buekens A, Sasco AJ. Polychlo-rinated biphenyls (Pcbs) in Africa: a review of environmental levels. *Environ Sci Pollut Res*. 2014;21:6278–6289.

Goncharoy A, Payuk M, Foushee HR, Carpenter DO. Blood pressure in relation to concen-trations of PCB congeners and chlorinated pesticides and Anniston Environmental Health Research Consortium. *Environmental Health Perspectives*. 2011;119(3):319-325.

Grandjean P, Gronlund C, Kjaer IM, Jensen TK, Sorensen N, Andersson AM, Juul A, Skakke-baek NE, Budtz-Jorgensen E, Weihe P. Reproductive hormone profile and pubertal devel-opment in 14-year-old boys prenatally exposed to polychlorinated biphenyls. *Reproductive Toxicology*. 2012;34:498–503.

Gray J, Dykema LD, Groetsch K. Health Consultation. Technical support document for a polychlorinated biphenyl reference dose (RfD) as a basis for fish consumption screening values (Fcsvs). Michigan Department of Community Health, Division of Environmental Health. November 1, 2012. ATSDR Region 5 Office.

Henry TR, DeVito MJ. Non-dioxin life Pcbs: Effects and consideration in ecological risk assessment. United States Environmental Protection Agency Experimental Toxicology Division National Health and Environmental Effects Research Laboratory Office of Research and Development NCEA-C-1340 ERASC-003 June 2003.

Herrick RF, Meeker JD, Altshul L. Serum PCB levels and congener profiles among teachers in PCB-containing schools: a pilot study. *Environmental Health*. 2011;10:56.

Hoogenboom R, Traag W, Fernandes A, Rose M. European developments following incidents with dioxins and Pcbs in the food and feed chain. *Food Control*. 2015;50:670-683.

Huetos O, Bartolome M, Aragones N, Cervantes-Amat M, Estaban M, Ruiz-Moraga R, Perez-Gomez B, Calvo E, Vila M, Castano A. Serum PCB levels in a representative sample of the Spanish adult population: The BIOAMBIENT.ES project. *Science of the Total Environment*. 2014;493:834–844.

Ibarluzea J, Alvarez-Pedrerol M, Guxens M, Basterrechea SMM, Lertxundi A, Etxeandia A, Goni F, Vioque J, Ballester F, Sunyer J. Sociodemographic, reproductive and dietary predictors of organochlorine compounds levels in pregnant women in Spain. *Chemosphere*. 2011;82:114–120.

Johansen EB, Fonnum F, Lausund PL, Walaas I, Baerland NE, Woien G, Sagvolden T. Behavioral changes following PCB 153 exposure in the spontaneously hypertensive rat – an animal model of attention-deficit/hyperactivity disorder. *Behavioral and Brain Functions*. 2014;10:1-19.

Kim D, Ryu HY, Lee JH, Lee JH, Lee YL, Kim HK, Jang DD, Kim HS, Yoon HS. Organochlorine pesticides and polychlorinated biphenyls in Korean human milk: Contamination levels and infant risk assessment, *Journal of Environmental Science and Health*, Part B: Pesticides, Food Contaminants, and Agricultural Wastes. 2013;48(4):243-250.

Kupferschmidt K. Dioxin scandal triggers food debate in Germany. *CMAJ*. 2011;183(4):E221-E222.

Lee DK, Lind L, Jacobs DR, Salihovic S, van Bavel Bert, Lind MP. Associations of persistent organic pollutants with abdominal obesity in the elderly: The Prospective Investigation of the Vasculature in Uppsala Seniors (PIVUS) study. *Environment International*. 2013;40:170–178.

Leong YH, Gan CY, Majid MIA. Dioxin-like polychlorinated biphenyls, polychlorinated dibenzop-dioxins, and polychlorinated dibenzofurans in seafood samples from Malaysia: Estimated human intake and associated risks. *Arch Environ Contam Toxicol*. 2014;67:21–28.

Lilienthal H, Heikkinen P, Andersson PL, van der Vene LTM, Viluksel M. Dopamine-dependent behavior in adult rats after perinatal exposure to purity-controlled polychlorinated biphenyl congeners (PCB52 andPCB180). *Toxicology Letters*. 2014;224:32-29.

Lin YS, Caffrey JL, Hsu PC, Chang MH, Faramawi MF, Lin JW. Environmental exposure to dioxin-like compounds and the mortality risk in the U.S. population. *International Journal of Hygiene and Environmental Health*. 2012;215:541–546.

Lind L, Penell J, Luttropp K, Nordfors L, Syvanen AC, Axelsson T, Salihovic S, van Bavel B, Fall T, Ingelsson E, Lind M. Global DNA hypermethylation is associated with high serum levels of persistent organic pollutants in an elderly population. *Environment International*. 2013;59:456–461.

Linnenbrink M. EPA Science in ACTION, Building a scientific foundation for sound environmental decisions. Polychlorinated biphenyls (Pcbs) research overview. *Communications*. 2013.

Luzardo OP, Almeida-Gonzalez M, Henriquez-Hernandez LA, Zumbado M, Alvarez-Leon

EE, Boada LD. Polychlorobiphenyls and organochlorine pesticides in conventional and organic brands of milk: Occurrence and dietary intake in the population of the Canary Islands (Spain). *Chemosphere.* 2012;88:307–315.

Malisch R, Kotz A. Dioxins and Pcbs in feed and food—Review from European perspective. *Science of the Total Environment.* 2014;491:2–10.

Mezzetta S, Cirlini M, Ceron P, Tecleanu A, Caligiani A, Palla G, Sansebastiano GE. Concentration of DL-Pcbs in fish from market of Parma city (north Italy): Estimated human intake. *Chemosphere.* 2011;82:1293–1300.

Morales E, Gascon M, Martinez D, Casas M, Ballester R, Rodriguez-Bernal CL, Ibarluzea J, Marina LS, Espada M, Goni F, Vizcaino E, Grimalt JO, Sunyer J. Associations between blood persistent organic pollutants and 25-hydroxyvitamin D3 in pregnancy. *Environment International.* 2013;57–58:34–41.

Morck TA, Erdmann SE, Long M, Mathiesen L, Nielsen F, Sierma VC, Bonefeld-Jorgensen EC, Knudsen LE. PCB Concentrations and Dioxin-like Activity in Blood Samples from Danish School Children and Their Mothers living in Urban and Rural Areas. *Basic & Clinical Pharmacology & Toxicology.* 2014;115:134–144.

Nakamoto M, Arisawa K, Uemura H, Katsuura S, Takami H, Sawachika F, Yamaguchi M, Juta T, Sakai T, Toda E, Mori K, Hasegawa Mn, Tanto M, Shima M, Sumiyoshi Y, Morinaga K, Kodama K, Suzuki T, Nagai M, Satoh H. Association between blood levels of Pcdds/Pcdfs/dioxin-like Pcbs and history of allergic and other diseases in the Japanese population. *Int Arch Occup Environ Health.* 2013;86:849–859.

Narbonne JF, Robertson LW. 7th International PCB Workshop: Chemical mixtures in a complex world. *Environ Sci Pollut Res.* 2014;21:6269–6275.

Ochiai S, Shimojo N, Yuka I, Watanabe M, Matsuno Y, Suzuki S, Kohno Y, Mori C. A pilot study for foetal exposure to multiple persistent organic pollutants and the development of infant atopic dermatitis in modern Japanese society. *Chemosphere.* 2014;94:48–52.

Park H, Park E, Chang YS. Ten-year time trend of dioxins in human serum obtained from metropolitan populations in Seoul, Korea. *Science of the Total Environment.* 2014;470:1338–1345.

Pavuk M, Olson JR, Sjodin A, Wolff P, Turner WE, Shelton C, Dutton ND, Bartell S. Serum concentrations of polychlorinated biphenyls (Pcbs) in participants of the Anniston Community Health Survey. *Science of the Total Environment.* 2014;473:286–297.

Pavuk M, Olson JR, Wattigney WA, Dutton ND, Sjodin A, Shelton C, Turner WE, Bartell SM. Predictors of serum polychlorinated biphenyl concentrations in Anniston residents. *Science of the Total Environment.* 2014;496:624–634.

Polychlorinated Biphenyls (Pcbs) TEACH Chemical Summary. USEPA, Toxicity and Exposure Assessment for Children's Health website 2011. Accessed July 27, 2015. Available at: https://archive.epa.gov/region5/teach/web/pdf/pcb_summary100809.pdf

Public Health Statement. Polychlorinated Biphenyls (PCBS) Division of Toxicology Nov 2002. Department of Health and Human Services, Public Health Agency for Toxic Substances and Disease Registry.

Robertson LW, Ludewig G. Polychlorinated Biphenyl (PCB) carcinogenicity with special emphasis on airborne Pcbs. *Gefahrst Reinhalt Luft.* 2011;71(1-2):25–32.

Ronn M, Lind L, van Bavel B, Salihovic S, Michaelsson K, Lind PM. Circulating levels of persistent organic pollutants associate in divergent ways to fat mass measured by DXA in humans. *Chemosphere.* 2011;85:335–343.

Roots O, Kivirantac H, Pitsi T, Rantakokko P, Ruokojarvi P, Simm M, Vokk R, Jarv L. Monitoring of polychlorinated dibenzo-p-dioxins, polychlorinated dibenzofurans, and polychlorinated biphenyls in Estonian food. *Proceedings of the Estonian Academy of Sciences.* 2011;60(3):193–200.

Roszko M, Szymczyk K, Jedrzejczak R. Influence of hen breeding type on PCDD/F, PCB & PBDE levels in eggs. *Science of the Total Environment.* 2014;487:279–289.

Rudge CVC, Sandanger T, Rollin HB, Calderon IMP, Volpato G, Silva JLP, Durate G, Neto CM, Sass N, Nakamura MU, Odland JO, Rudge MVC. Levels of selected persistent organic pollutants in blood from delivering women in seven selected areas of São Paulo State, Brazil. *Environment International.* 2012;40;162–169.

Rylander C, Lund E, Froyland L, Sandanger TM. Predictors of PCP, OH-Pcbs, Pcbs and chlorinated pesticides in a general female Norwegian population. *Environment International.* 2012;43:13–20.

Salihovic S, Lampa E, Lindstrom G, Lind L, Lind PM, van Bavel B. Circulating levels of Persistent Organic Pollutants (POPs) among elderly men and women from Sweden: Results from the Prospective Investigation of the Vasculature in Uppsala Seniors (PIVUS). *Environment International.* 2013;44:59–67.

Schettgen T, Alt A, Preim D, Keller D, Kraus T. Biological monitoring of indoor-exposure to dioxin-like and non-dioxin-like polychlorinated biphenyls (PCB) in a public building. *Toxicology Letters.* 2012;213:116-121.

Schug TT, Janesick A, Blumberg B, Jeindel JJ. Endocrine disrupting chemicals and disease susceptibility. *Journal of Steroid Biochemistry & Molecular Biology.* 2011;127:204– 215.

Senthilkumar PK, Robertson LW, Ludewig G. PCB153 reduces telomerase activity and telomere length in immortalized human skin keratinocytes (HaCaT) but not in human foreskin keratinocytes (NFK). *Toxicology and Applied Pharmacology.* 2012;259:115–123.

Serdar B, LeBlanc WG, Norris JM, Dickinson LM. Potential effects of polychlorinated biphenyls (PCBs) and selected organochlorine pesticides (Ocps) on immune cells and blood biochemistry measures: a cross-sectional assessment of the NHANES 2003-2004 data. *Environmental Health.* 2014;13:114-126.

Serveev AV, Carpenter DO. Increase in metabolic syndrome-related hospitalizations in relation to environmental sources of persistent organic pollutants. *Int. J. Environ. Res. Public Health.* 2011;8:762-776.

Storelli MM, Barone G, Perrone VG, Giacominelli-Stuffler R. Polychlorinated biphenyls (PCBs), dioxins and furans (PCDD/Fs): Occurrence in fishery products and dietary intake. *Food Chemistry.* 2011;127:1648–1652.

Tait S, La Rocca C, Mantovani A. Exposure of human fetal penile cells to different PCB mixtures: transcriptome analysis points to diverse modes of interference on external genitalia programming. *Reproductive Toxicology.* 2011;32:1–14.

Turnkvist A, Glynn A, Aune M, Darnerud PO, Ankarbert EH. PCDD/F, PCB, PBDE, HBCD and chlorinated pesticides in a Swedish market basket from 2005 – Levels and dietary intake estimations. *Chemosphere.* 2011;83:193–199.

Wens B, Boevera PD, Maes M, Hollanders K, Schoeters G. Transcriptomics identifies differences between ultrapure non-dioxin-like polychlorinated biphenyls (PCBs) and dioxin-like PCB126 in cultured peripheral blood mononuclear cells. *Toxicology.* 2011;287:113– 123.

Winneke G, Ranft U, Wittsiepe J, Kasper-Sonnenberg M, Furst P, Kramer U, Seitner G, Wilhelm M. Behavioral sexual dimorphism in school-age children and early developmental exposure to dioxins and Pcbs: A follow-up study of the Duisburg Cohort. *Environ Health Perspect.* 2014;122:292-298.

Xing GH, Liang Y, Chen LX, Wua SC, Wong MH. Exposure to PCBs, through inhalation, dermal contact and dust ingestion at Taizhou, China – A major site for recycling transformers. *Chemosphere.* 2011;83:605–611.

Xinghui SW, Yang L, Liu H. Distribution, source and risk assessment of polychlorinated biphenyls (Pcbs) in urban soils of Beijing, China. *Chemosphere.* 2011;82:732–738.

CHAPTER 5 – PLASTICS FOR DURABILITY & TRANSPARENCY: PHTHALATES
ATSDR Public Health Statement. This Public Health Statement is the summary chapter from the Toxicological Profile for Di(2- ethylhexyl) phthalate (DEHP) Department of Health and Human Services, Public Health Service Agency for Toxic Substances and Disease Registry Public Health Statement. Di(2-ethylhexyl)phthalate (DEHP) CAS#: 117-81-7

Buckley JP, Palmieri RT, Matuszewski JM, Herring AH, Baird DD, Hartmann KE, Hoppin JA. Consumer product exposures associated with urinary phthalate levels in pregnant women. *Journal of Exposure Science and Environmental Epidemiology.* 2012;22:468-475.

Buttke DE, Sircar K, Martin C. Exposures to endocrine-disrupting chemicals and age of menarche in adolescent girls in NHANES (2003–2008). *Environ Health Perspect.* 2012;120:1613–1618.

Crinnion WJ. Toxic Effects of the Easily Avoidable Phthalates and Parabens. *Altern Med Rev.* 2010;15(3):190-196.

DiGangi J, Schettler T, Cobbing M, Rossi M. Aggregate Exposures to phthalates in humans. Health Care Without Harm. July 2002.

Early Life Exposure to Phthalates and Breast Cancer Risk in Later Years. Fact Sheet on Phthalates. 11/7/07. Breast Cancer & The Environment Research Centers.

Goen T, Dobler L, Koschorreck J, Muller J, Wiesmuller GA, Drexler H, Kolossa-Gehring M. Trends of the internal phthalate exposure of young adults in Germany—Follow-up of a retrospective human biomonitoring study. *International Journal of Hygiene and Environmental Health.* 2011;215:36–45.

Guerranti C, Sbordoni I, Fanello EL, Borghini F, Corsi I, Focardi SE. Levels of phthalates in human milk samples from central Italy. *Microchemical Journal.* 2013;107:178–181.

Guo Y, Wu Q, Kannan K. Phthalate metabolites in urine from China, and implications for human exposures. *Environment International.* 2011;37:893–898.

Healthy Building Website. 2016. Accessed March 28, 2016. Available at: **http://healthybuilding. net/.**

Hsu NY, Lee CC, Wang JY, Li YC, Chang HW, Chen CY, Bornehag CG, Wu PC, Sundell J, Su HJ. Predicted risk of childhood allergy, asthma, and reported symptoms using measured phthalate exposure in dust and urine. *Indoor Air.* 2012;22:186–199.

International Chemical Secretariat, ChemSec. In focus: Endocrine disrupting chemicals. Phthalates. The SIN List. 2015. Accessed March 28, 2016. Available at: **http://chemsec.org/ what-we-do/sin-list.**

Joensen UN, Frederiksen H, Jensen MB, Lauritsen MP, Olesen IA, Lassen TH, Andersson AM, Jorgensen N. Phthalate excretion pattern and testicular function: a study of 881 healthy Danish Men. *Environ Health Perspect.* 2013;120:1397–1403.

Johnson S, Saikia N, Sahu R. Phthalates in toys available in Indian market. *Bull Environ Contam Toxicol.* 2011;86:621–626.

Juhasz MLW, Marmur ES. A review of selected chemical additives in cosmetic products. *Dermatologic Therapy.* 2014;27:317–322.

Jurewicz J, Radwan M, Sobala W, Ligocka D, Radwan P, Bochenek M, Hawula W, Jakubowski L, Hanke W. Human urinary phthalate metabolites level and main semen parameters, sperm chromatin structure, sperm aneuploidy and reproductive hormones. *Reproductive Toxicology.* 2013;42:232–241.

Lin LC, Wang SL, Chang YC, Huang PC, Cheng JT, Su PH, Liao PC. Associations between maternal phthalate exposure and cord sex hormones in human infants. *Chemosphere.* 2011;83:1192–1199.

Lin S, Ku HY, Su PH, Chen JW, Huang PC, Angerer J, Wang SL. Phthalate exposure in pregnant women and their children in central Taiwan. *Chemosphere.* 2011;82:947–955.

Liu L, Bao H, Liu F, Zhang J, Shen H. Phthalates exposure of Chinese reproductive age couples and its effect on male semen quality, a primary study. *Environment International.* 2012;42:78–83.

Parlett LE, Calafat AM, Swan SH. Women's exposure to phthalates in relation to use of personal care products. *J Expo Sci Environ Epidemiol.* 2013;23(2):197–206.

Phthalates and Parabens Measured on the Metametrix Profile. Metametrix Clinical Laboratory, Phthalates & Parabens Profile Interpretive Guide. Duluth, GA

Phthalates. TEACH Chemical Summary. U.S. EPA, Toxicity and Exposure Assessment for Children's Health. Last revised 10/10/2007.

Pilka T, Petrovicova I, Kolena B, Zatko T, Trnovec T. Relationship between variation of seasonal temperature and extent of occupational exposure to phthalates. *Environ Sci Pollut Res.* 2015;22:434–440.

Polanska K, Ligocka D, Sobala W, Hanke W. Phthalate exposure and child development: The Polish Mother and Child Cohort Study. *Early Human Development.* 2014;90:477–485.

Schecter A, Lorber M, Guo Y, Wu Q, Yun SE, Kannan K, Hommel M, Imran N, Hynan LS, Cheng D, Colacino JA, Birnbaum LS. Phthalate concentrations and dietary exposure from food purchased in New York State. *Environ Health Perspect.* 2013;121:473–479.

Serrano SE, Braun J, Trasande L, Dills R, Sathyanarayana S. Phthalates and diet: a review of the food monitoring and epidemiology data. *Environmental Health.* 2014;13:43. http://www.ehjournal.net/content/13/1/43

Serrano SE, Karr CJ, Seixas NS, Nguyen RHN, Barrett ES, Janssen S, Redmon B, Swan SH, Sathyanarayana S. Dietary phthalate exposure in pregnant women and the impact of consumer practices. *Int. J. Environ. Res. Public Health.* 2014;11:6193-6215.

Shiue I. Higher urinary heavy metal, phthalate, and arsenic but not parabens concentrations in people with high blood pressure, U.S. NHANES, 2011–2012. *Int. J. Environ. Res. Public Health* 2014;11:5989-5999.

Singh S, Li SSL. Phthalates: Toxicogenomics and inferred human diseases. *Genomics.* 2011;97:148–157.

Tang-Péronard JL, Andersen HR, Jensen TK, Heitmann BL. Endocrine-disrupting chemicals and obesity development in humans: A review. *Obesity Reviews.* 2011;12:622–636.

Teitelbaum SL, Mervish N, Moshier EL, Vangeepuram N, Galvez MP, Calafat AM, Silva MJ, Brenner BL, Wolff MS. Associations between phthalate metabolite urinary concentrations and body size measures in New York City children. *Environmental Research.* 2013;112:186–193.

Toshima H, Suzuki Y, Imai K, Yoshinaga J, Shiraishi H, Mizumoto Y, Hatakeyama S, Onohara C, Tokuoka S. Endocrine disrupting chemicals in urine of Japanese male partners of subfertile couples: A pilot study on exposure and semen quality. *International Journal of Hygiene and Environmental Health.* 2012;215:502–506.

Tranfo G, Papaleo B, Caporossi L, Capanna S, De Rosa M, Pigini D, Corsetti F, Paci E. Urinary metabolite concentrations of phthalate metabolites in Central Italy healthy volunteers determined by a validated HPLC/MS/MS analytical method. *International Journal of Hygiene and*

Environmental Health. 2013;216:481–485.

What are phthalates? Alaska Community Action on Toxics. Accessed March 29, 2016. Available at: http://www.akaction.org/wp-content/uploads/2013/03/Phthalates_ACAT2.pdf.

Whyatt RM, Liu X, Rauh VA, Calafat AM, Just AC, Hoepner L, Diaz D, Quinn J, Adibi J, Perera FP, Factor-Litvak P. Maternal prenatal urinary phthalate metabolite concentrations and child mental, psychomotor, and behavioral development at 3 years of age. *Environ Health Perspect.* 2012;120:290–295.

Xu Y, Liu Z, Park Jinsoo, Clausen PA, Benning JL, Little JC. Measuring and predicting the emission rate of phthalate plasticizer from vinyl flooring in a specially-designed chamber. *Environ. Sci. Technol.* 2012;46:12534-12541.

CHAPTER 6 – YET ONE MORE PLASTICS CHEMICAL: BISPHENOL A (BPA)

Arnold SM, Clark KE, Staples CA, Klecka GM, Dimond SS, Caspers N, Hentges SG. Relevance of drinking water as a source of human exposure to bisphenol A. *Journal of Exposure Science and Environmental Epidemiology.* 2013;23:137-144.

Bisphenol A. National Institute of Environmental Health Sciences website. Accessed March 9, 2016. Available at: http://www.niehs.nih.gov/health/topics/agents/sya-bpa/ .

BPA Coats Cash Register Receipts. The Environmental Working Group website. 2015. Accessed March 10, 2016. Available at: http://www.ewg.org/research/bpa-in-store-receipts.

Brien MA, Reig-Viader R, Cabero L, Toran N, Martinez F, Roig I, Calde MG. Gene expression is altered after bisphenol A exposure in human fetal oocytes in vitro. *Molecular Human Reproduction.* 2012;18(4):71–183.

Chena M, Tanga R, Fu G, Xua B, Zhud P, Qiao S, Chena X, Xua B, Qina Y, Lu C, Hange B, Xia Y, Wanga X. Association of exposure to phenols and idiopathic male infertility. *Journal of Hazardous Materials.* 2013;250–251:115–121.

Cladiere M, Gasperi J, Lorgeoux C, Bonhomme C, Rocher V, Tassin. B. Alkylphenolic compounds and bisphenol A contamination within a heavily urbanized area: case study of Paris. *Environ Sci Pollut Res.* 2013;20:2973–2983.

Colin A, Bach C, Rosin C, Munoz JF, Dauchy X. Is drinking water a major route of human exposure to alkylphenol and bisphenol contaminants in France? *Arch Environ Contam Toxicol.* 2014;66:86–99.

Dupuis A, Migeot V, Cariot A, Albouy-Llaty M, Legube B, Rabouan S. Quantification of bisphenol A, 353-nonylphenol and their chlorinated derivatives in drinking water treatment plants. *Environ Sci Pollut Res.* 2012;19:4193–4205.

Esteban S, Gorga M, Gonzalez-Alonso S, Petrovic M, Barcelo D, Valcarcel Y. Monitoring endocrine disrupting compounds and estrogenic activity in tap water from Central Spain. *Environ Sci Pollut Res.* 2014;21:9297–9310.

Geens T, Aaerts D, Berthot C, Bourguignon JP, Goeyens L, Lecomte P, Maghuin-Register G, Pironnet AM, Pussemier L, Scippo ML, Van Loco J, Covaci A. A review of dietary and non-dietary exposure to bisphenol-A. *Food and Chemical Toxicology.* 2012;50:3725–3740.

Geens T, Goeyens L, Kannan K, Neels H, Covaci A. Levels of bisphenol-A in thermal paper receipts from Belgium and estimation of human exposure. *Science of the Total Environment.* 2012;435–436:30–33.

Gong H, Zhang X, Cheng B, Sun Y, Li C, et al. Bisphenol A accelerates toxic amyloid formation of human islet amyloid polypeptide: a possible link between bisphenol A exposure and type 2 diabetes. 2013. PLoS ONE 8(1): e54198. doi:10.1371/journal.pone.0054198

Guart A. Bono-Blay F, Borrell A, Lacorte S. Migration of plasticizers phthalates, bisphenol A and alkylphenols from plastic containers and evaluation of risk. *Food Additives & Contaminants.* 2011;28(5):676-685.

Huang YQ, Wong CKC, Zheng JS, Bouwman H, Barra R, Wahlstrom B, Neretin L, Wong MH. Bisphenol A (BPA) in China: A review of sources, environmental levels, and potential human health impacts. *Environment International.* 2012;42:91–99.

Li X, Ying GG, Zhao JL, Chen ZF, Lai HJ, Su HC. 4-Nonylphenol, bisphenol-A and triclosan levels in human urine of children and students in China, and the effects of drinking these bottled materials on the levels. *Environment International.* 2013;52:81–86.

Liao C, Kannan K. Concentrations and profiles of bisphenol A and other bisphenol analogues in foodstuffs from the United States and their implications for human exposure. *J. Agric. Food Chem.* 2013;61:4655-4662.

Liao C, Kannan K. Widespread occurrence of bisphenol A in paper and paper products: implications for human exposure. *Environ. Sci. Technol.* 2011;45:9372–9379.

Liao C, Liu F, Guo Y, Moon HB, Nakata H, Wu Q, Kannan K. Occurrence of eight bisphenol analogues in indoor dust from the United States and several Asian countries: implications for human exposure. *Environ. Sci. Technol.* 2012;46:9138-9145.

Liu J, Yu P, Qian W, Li Y, Zhao J, et al. Perinatal bisphenol A exposure and adult glucose homeostasis: identifying critical windows of exposure. PLoS ONE 8(5): e64143. doi:10.1371/journal.pone.0064143

Loganathan SN, Kannan K. Occurrence of Bisphenol A in indoor dust from two locations in the Eastern United States and implications for human exposures. *Arch Environ Contam Toxicol.* 2011;61:68–73.

Lu SY, Chang WJ, Sojinu SO, Ni HG. Bisphenol A in supermarket receipts and its exposure to humans in Shenzhen, China. *Chemosphere.* 2013;92:1190–1194.

Michalowicz J. Bisphenol A – sources, toxicity and biotransformation. *Environmental Toxicology and Pharmacology.* 2014;37:738-758.

Migeot V, Dupuis A, Cariot A, Albouy-Llaty M, Pierre F, Rabouan S. Bisphenol A and its chlorinated derivatives in human colostrum. *Environ. Sci. Technol.* 2013;47:13791-13797.

Moghadam ZA, Mirlohi M, Pourzamani H, Malekpour A. Bisphenol A in "BPA free" baby feeding bottles. *J Res Med Sci.* 2012;17(11):1089–1091.

Nahar MS, Liao C, Kannan K, Dolinoy DC. Fetal liver bisphenol A concentrations and biotransformation gene expression reveal variable exposure and altered capacity for metabolism in humans. *J Biochem Mol Toxicol.* 2013;27:116–123.

Pirard C, Sagot C, Deville M, Dubois N, Charlier C. Urinary levels of bisphenol A, triclosan and 4-nonylphenol in a general Belgian population. *Environment International.* 2012;48:78–83.

Renz L, Volz C, Michanowicz D, Ferrar K, Christian C, Lenzner D, El-Hefnawy T. A study of parabens and bisphenol A in surface water and fish brain tissue from the Greater Pittsburgh Area. *Ecotoxicology.* 2013;22:632–641.

Rochester JR. Bisphenol A and human health: a review of the literature. *Reproductive Toxicology.* 2013;42:132-155.

Rubin JR. Bisphenol A: An endocrine disruptor with widespread exposure and multiple effects. *Journal of Steroid Biochemistry & Molecular Biology.* 2011;127:27– 34.

Sathyanarayana S. Alcedo G, Saelens BE, Zhou C, Dills RL, Yu J, Lanphear B. Unexpected results in a randomized dietary trial to reduce phthalate and bisphenol A exposures. *Journal of Exposure Science and Environmental Epidemiology.* 2013;23:378-384.

Tiwari D, Kambele J, Chilgunde S, Patil P, Maru G, Kawle D, Bhartiya U, Joseph L, Vanage G. Clastogenic and mutagenic effects of bisphenol A: an endocrine disruptor. *Mutation Research.*

2012;743:83–90.

Turnage BF. Fetal and infant exposure to bisphenol A. *International Journal of Childbirth Education*. 2013;28(4):32-33.

Vandenberg LN. Exposure to bisphenol A in Canada: invoking the precautionary principle. *CMAJ*. 2011;183(11):1265-1271.

CHAPTER 7 – SANITIZERS

TRICLOSAN

Bedoux G, Roig B. Thomas O, Dupont V, Le Bot B. Occurrence and toxicity of antimicrobial triclosan and by-products in the environment. *Environ Sci Pollut Res*. 2011;19:1044–1065.

Bergstrom KG. Update on antibacterial soaps: The FDA takes a second look at triclosans. *Journal of Drugs in Dermatology*. 2014;13(4):501-503.

Brausch JM, Rand GM. A review of personal care products in the aquatic environment: environmental concentrations and toxicity. *Chemosphere*. 2011;82:1518–1532.

Chen M, Tanga R, Fu Guangbo, Su B, Zhud P, Qiao S, Chen X, Su B, Qin Y, Lu C. Hange B, Xia Y, Wang X. Association of exposure to phenols and idiopathic male infertility. *Journal of Hazardous Materials*. 2013;250–251:115–121.

Clayton EMR, Todd M, Dowd JB, Aiello AE. The impact of bisphenol A and triclosan on immune parameters in the U. S. population. NHANES 2003-2006. *Environ Health Perspect*. 2011;119:390-396.

Dann AB, Hontela A. Triclosan: environmental exposure, toxicity and mechanisms of action. *J. Appl. Toxicol*. 2011;31:285–311.

European Commission Scientific Committee on Consumer Safety. Opinion on triclosan antimicrobial resistance. June 2010.

Geens T, Neels H, Covac A. Distribution of bisphenol-A, triclosan and n-nonylphenol in human adipose tissue, liver and brain. *Chemosphere*. 2012;87:796–802.

Halden RU. On the need and speed of regulating triclosan and triclocarban in the United States. *Environ. Sci. Technol*. 2014;48:3603-3611.

Honkisz E, Ziega-Przybylska D. Wojtowicz AK. The effect of triclosan on hormone secretion and viability of human choriocarcinoma JEG-3 cells. *Reproductive Toxicology*. 2012;34:385-392.

Lankester J, Patel C, Cullen MR, Ley C, Parsonnet J. Urinary triclosan is associated with elevated body mass index in NHANES. PLoS ONE 2013;8(11): e80057. doi:10.1371/journal.pone.0080057

Li X, Ying GG, Zhao JL, Chen ZF, Lai HJ, Su HC. 4-Nonylphenol, bisphenol-A and triclosan levels in human urine of children and students in China, and the effects of drinking these bottled materials on the levels. *Environment International*. 2013;52:81–86.

National Drug Code Directory. The United States Food and Drug Administration website. Accessed March 7, 2016. Available at: http://www.accessdata.fda.gov/scripts/cder/ndc/default.cfm

Perez AL, De Sylor MA, Slocombe AJ, Lew MG, Unice KM, Donovan EP. Triclosan occurrence in freshwater systems in the United States (1999–2012): a meta-analysis. *Environmental Toxicology and Chemistry*. 2013;32(7):1479–1487.

Pirard C, Sagot C, Deville M, Dubois N, Charlier C. Urinary levels of bisphenol A, triclosan and 4-nonylphenol in a general Belgian population. *Environment International*. 2012;48:78–83.

Preliminary Assessment. Triclosan. Chemical Abstracts Service Registry Number 3380-34-5. Health Canada, Environment Canada. March 2012.

Pycke BFG, Geer LA, Dalloul M, Abulafia O, Jenck AM, Halden RU. Human fetal exposure to Triclosan and triclocarban in an urban population from Brooklyn, New York. *Environ. Sci. Technol.* 2014;48:8831–8838.

Savage JH, Matsui EC, Wood RA, Keet CA. Urinary levels of triclosan and parabens are associated with aeroallergen and food sensitization. *J Allergy Clin Immunol.* 2012;130:453-460.

The Environmental Working Group's Guide to Triclosan. Available at: http://www.ewg.org/sites/default/files/EWG_triclosanguide.pdf

Toms LML, Allmyr M, Mueller JF, Adolfsson-Erici M, McLachlan M, Murby J, Harden FA. Triclosan in individual human milk samples from Australia. *Chemosphere.* 2011;85:1682–1686.

Triclosan *White Paper prepared by The Alliance for the Prudent Use of Antibiotics (APUA)* January 2011.

Yueh MF, Tanguchi K, Chen S, Evans RM, Hammock BD, Karin M, Tukey RH. The commonly used antimicrobial additive triclosan is a liver tumor promoter. *PNAS.* 2014;111(48):17200–17205.

CHAPTER 8 – SURFACTANTS

4-NONYLPHENOL

Balakrishnan B, Thorstensen E, Ponnampalam A, Mitchell MD. Passage of 4-nonylphenol across the human placenta. *Placenta.* 2011;32:788-792.

Bontje D, Hermens J, Vermeire T, Damstra T. International Programme on Chemical Safety Integrated Risk Assessment: Nonylphenol. 12/04.

Carlisle J, Chan D, Painter P, Wu L. Toxicological Profile for Nonylphenol. September 2009. Integrated Risk Assessment Branch, Office of Environmental Health Hazard Assessment, California Environmental Protection Agency.

Chrostowski P. Fact Sheet: Alkylphenols in biosolids. March 2002

Cladiere M, Gasperi J, Lorgeoux C, Bonhomme C, Rocher V, Tassin B. Alkylphenolic compounds and bisphenol A contamination within a heavily urbanized area: case study of Paris. *Environ Sci Pollut Res.* 2013;20:2973–2983.

European Union Risk Assessment Report. 4-nonylphenol (branched) and nonylphenol. EINECS Nos: 284-325-5, 246-672-0. Volume 10. 2nd Priority List. 2002, United Kingdom.

Geens T, Neels H, Covac A. Distribution of bisphenol-A, triclosan and n-nonylphenol in human adipose tissue, liver and brain. *Chemosphere.* 2012;87:96–802.

Gyllenhammar I, Glynn A, Darnerud PO, Lignell S, van Delft R, Aue M. 4-Nonylphenol and bisphenol A in Swedish food and exposure in Swedish nursing women. *Environment International.* 2012;43:21–28.

Lu T, Zhao XE, Zhu S, Qu F, Song C, You J, Suo Y. Determination of bisphenol A, 4-octylphenol, and 4-nonylphenol in soft drinks and dairy products by ultrasound-assisted dispersive liquid–liquid microextraction combined with derivatization and high-performance liquid chromatography with fluorescence detection. *J. Sep. Sci.* 2014;37:2757–2763.

Manente L, Sellitti A, Lucariello A, Laforgia V, De Falco M, De Luca A. Effects of 4-nonylphenol on proliferation of AGS gastric cells. *Cell Prolif.* 2011;44:477–485.

Munaron D, Tapie N, Budzinski H, Andral B, Gonzalea JL. Pharmaceuticals, alkylphenols and pesticides in Mediterranean coastal waters: results from a pilot survey using passive samplers. *Estuarine, Coastal and Shelf Science.* 2012;114:82-92.

Pirard C, Sagot C, Deville M, Dubois N. Charlier C. Urinary levels of bisphenol A, triclosan and 4-nonylphenol in a general Belgian population. *Environment International.* 2012;48:78–83.

Suen JL, Hsu SH, Hung CH, Chao YS, Lee CL, Lin CY, Weng TH, Yu HS, Huang SK. A common environmental pollutant, 4-nonylphenol, promotes allergic lung inflammation in a murine model of asthma. *Allergy.* 2013;68:780–787.

Suen JL, Hung CH, Yu HS, Huang SK. Alkylphenols and potential modulators of the allergic response. *Kaohsiung Journal of Medical Sciences.* 2012;28:S43-S48.

U.S. Environmental Protection Agency 8/18/2010. Nonylphenol (NP) and Nonylphenol Ethoxylates (NPEs) Action Plan.

Yen CH, Sun CK, Leu S, Wallace CG, Lin YC, Chang LT, Chen YL, Tsa TH, Kao YG, Shao PL, Hsieh CY, Chen YT, Yip HK. Continuing exposure to low-dose nonylphenol aggravates adenine-induced chronic renal dysfunction and role of rosuvastatin therapy. *Journal of Translational Medicine.* 2012;10:147. DOI: 10.1186/1479-5876-10-147.

Zhang HY, Xue WY, Li YY, Ma Y, Zhua YS, Huo WQ, Xu B, Xia W, Xu SQ. Perinatal exposure to 4-nonylphenol affects adipogenesis in first and second generation rats offspring. *Toxicology Letters.* 2014;225:325–332.

CHAPTER 9 – ANTIBACTERIALS IN PERSONAL CARE PRODUCTS: PARABENS

Barr L, Metaxas G, Harbach AJ, Savoy LA, Darbre PD. Measurement of paraben concentrations in human breast tissue at serial locations across the breast from axilla to sternum. *J. Appl. Toxicol.* 2012;32:219–232.

Crinnion WJ. Toxic effects of the easily avoidable phthalates and parabens. *Altern Med Rev.* 2010;15(3):190-196.

Darbre PD, Harvey PW. Parabens can enable hallmarks and characteristics of cancer in human breast epithelial cells: a review of the literature with reference to new exposure data and regulatory status. *J. Appl. Toxicol.* 2014;34:925–938.

Harvey PW, Everett DJ. Parabens detection in different zones of the human breast: consideration of source and implications of findings. *J. Appl. Toxicol.* 2012;32:305–309.

Ma D, Chen L, Zhu X, Li F, Liu C, Liu R. Assessment of combined antiandrogenic effects of binary parabens mixtures in a yeast-based reporter assay. *Environ Sci Pollut Res.* 2014;21:6482–6494.

Ma WL, Wang L, Guo Y, Liu LY, Qi H, Zhu NZ, Gao CJ, Li YF, Kannan K. Urinary concentrations of parabens in Chinese young adults: Implications for human exposure. *Arch Environ Contam Toxicol.* 2013;65:611–618.

Makaji E, Raha S, Wade MG, Holloway AC. Effect of environmental contaminants on beta cell function. *International Journal of Toxicology.* 2011;30(4):410-418.

Parabens. CDC Environmental Health, May 2010.

Pazourekova S, Hojerova J, Klimova Z, Lucova M. Dermal absorption and hydrolysis of methylparaben in different vehicles through intact and damaged skin: Using a pig-ear model in vitro. *Food and Chemical Toxicology.* 2013;59:754–765.

Philippat C, Wolff MS, Calafat AM, Ye X, Bausell R, Meadows M, Stone J, Slama R, Engel SM. Prenatal exposure to environmental phenols: concentrations in amniotic fluid and variability in urinary concentrations during pregnancy. *Environ Health Perspect.* 2013;121:1225-1231.

Ryu J, Oh J, Snyder SA, Yoon Y. Determination of micropollutants in combined sewer overflows and their removal in a wastewater treatment plant (Seoul, South Korea). *Environ Monit Assess.* 2014;186:3239-3251.

Scientific Committee on Consumer Safety. SCCS Opinion on Parabens. Updated request for a scientific opinion on propyl- and butylparaben. European Commission. May 2013.

Smith KW, Braun JM, Williams PL, Ehrlich S, Correia KF, Calafat AM, Ye X, Ford J, Keller M, Meeker JD, Hauser R. Predictors and variability of urinary paraben concentrations in men and women, including before and during pregnancy. *Environ Health Perspect.* 2012;120(11):1538-1543.

Smith KW, Souter I, Dimitriadis I, Ehrlich S, Williams PL, Calafat AM, Hauser R. Urinary paraben concentrations and ovarian aging among women from a fertility center. *Environ Health Perspect.* 2013;121:1299-1305.

Yamamoto H, Tamura I, Hirata Y, Kato J, Kagota K, Katsuki S, Yamamoto A, Kagami Y, Tatarazako N. Aquatic toxicity and ecological risk assessment of seven parabens: Individual and additive approach. *Science of the Total Environment.* 2011;410: 102–111.

Yang P, Ren H, Qui H, Kiu X, Jiang S. Determination of four trace preservatives in street food by ionic liquid-based dispersive liquid–liquid micro-extraction. *Chemical Papers.* 2011;65(6):747–753.

Yazar K, Johnsson S, Lind ML, Moman A, Liden C. Preservatives and fragrances in selected consumer-available cosmetics and detergents. *Contact Dermatitis.* 2010;64:265–272.

CHAPTER 10 – DETOXIFICATION

Alves A, Kucharska A, Erratico C, Xu F, Hond ED, Koppen G, Vanermen G, Covaci A, Voorspoels S. Human biomonitoring of emerging pollutants through non-invasive matrices: state of the art and future potential. *Anal Bioanal Chem.* 2014;406:4063–4088.

Arrebola JP, Fernandez MF, Molina-Molina JM, Olmedob PM, Expositod J, Olea N. Predictors of the total effective xenoestrogen burden (TEXB) in human adipose tissue. A pilot study. *Reproductive Toxicology.* 2012;33:45-52.

Bare facts of the sauna. This is Finland website. 2009. Accessed August 4, 2015. Available at: http://finland.fi/life-society/bare-facts-of-the-sauna/.

Berman T, Amitai Y, Almog S, Richter ED. Human biomonitoring in Israel: Past, present, future. *International Journal of Hygiene and Environmental Health.* 2012;215:138-141.

Body burden: The pollution in newborns. The Environmental Working Group website. 2015. Accessed August 5, 2015. Available at: http://www.ewg.org/research/body-burden-pollution-newborns.

Choi JJ, Eum SY, Rampersaud E, Daunert S, Abreu MT, Toborek M. Exercise attenuates PCB-induced changes in the mouse gut microbiome. *Environmental Health Perspectives.* 2013;121(6):725-731.

Clostre F, Letourmy P, Thuries L, Lesueur-Jannoyer M. Effect of home food processing on chlordecone (organochlorine) content in vegetables. *Science of the Total Environment.* 2014;490:1044-1050.

Crinnion WJ. Chlorinated pesticides: Threats to health and importance of detection. *Altern Med Rev.* 2009;14(4):347-359.

Crinnion WJ. Sauna as a valuable clinical tool for cardiovascular, autoimmune, toxicant induced and other chronic health problems. *Altern Med Rev.* 2011;16(3)_215-225.

Cruciferous vegetables. Linus Pauling Institute. Oregon State University website. 2015. Accessed August 4, 2015. Available at: http://lpi.oregonstate.edu/mic/food-beverages/cruciferous-vegetables.

Devier MH, Mazellier P, Aissa SA, Budzinski H. New challenges in environmental analytical chemistry: Identification of toxic compounds in complex mixtures. *C.R. Chimie.* 2011;14:766-779.

Falkowska L, Reindl AR, Szumilo E, Kwasniak J, Staniszewska M, Beldowska M, Lewandowska A, Krause K. Mercury and chlorinated pesticides on the highest level of the food web as exemplified by herring from the southern Baltic and African penguins from the zoo. *Water*

Air Soil Pollut. 2013;224:1549-1563.

Foods that fight cancer. American Institute for Cancer Research website. 2015. Accessed August 4, 2015. Available at: http://preventcancer.aicr.org/site/PageServer?pagename=foodsthat-fightcancer_garlic.

Gennings C, Ellis R, Ritter JK. Linking empirical estimates of body burden of environmental chemicals and wellness using NHANES data. *Environment International*. 2012;39:56-65.

Genuis SJ. Sensitivity-related illness: the escalating pandemic of allergy, food intolerance and chemical sensitivity. *Science of the Total Environment*. 2010;408(24):6047–6061.

Genuis SJ. Elimination of persistent toxicants from the human body. *Human and Experimental Toxicology*. 2011;30(1):3-18.

Genuis SJ, Beesoon S, Birkholz D. Biomonitoring and elimination of perfluorinated compounds and polychlorinated biphenyls through perspiration: Blood, urine, and sweat study. *ISRN Toxicology*. 2013, Article ID 483832, 7 pages. http://dx.doi.org/10.1155/2013/483832.

Genuis SJ, Beesoon S, Lobo RA, Birkholz D. Human elimination of phthalate compounds: Blood, urine, and sweat (BUS) study. *The Scientific World Journal*. Volume 2012, Article ID 615068, 10 pages. doi:10.1100/2012/615068

Genuis SJ, Curtis L, Birkholz D. Gastrointestinal elimination of perfluorinated compounds using cholestyramine and chlorella pyrenoidosa. *ISRN Toxicology*. 2013, Article ID 657849, 8 pages. http://dx.doi.org/10.1155/2013/657849.

Genuis SJ, Sears ME, Schwalfenberg G, Hope J, Bernoft R. Clinical detoxification: Elimination of persistent toxicants from the human body. *The Scientific World Journal*. Volume 2013, Article ID 238347, 3 pages. http://dx.doi.org/10.1155/2013/238347

Hong NS, Kim KS, Lee IK, Lind PM, Lind L, Jacobs DR, Lee DH. The association between obesity and mortality in the elderly differs by serum concentrations of persistent organic pollutants: a possible explanation for the obesity paradox. *International Journal of Obesity*. 2012;36:1170-1175.

Jandacek RJ, Genuis SJ. An assessment of the intestinal lumen as a site for intervention in reducing body burdens of organochlorine compounds. *The Scientific World Journal*. Volume 2013, Article ID 205621, 10 pages. http://dx.doi.org/10.1155/2013/205621

Jurewicz J, Polanska K, Hanke W. Exposure to widespread environmental toxicants and children's cognitive development and behavioral problems. *Int J Occup Med Environ Health*. 2013;26(2):185-204.

Klein AV, Kiat H. Detox diets for toxin elimination and weight management: a critical review of the evidence. *J Hum Nutr Diet*. 2014. doi: 10.1111/jhn.12286.

Metabolic detoxification. LifeExtension website. 2015. Accessed August 3, 2015. Available at http://www.lef.org/Protocols/Metabolic-Health/Metabolic-Detoxification/Page-01.

Metametrix Clinical Laboratory, Phthalates & Parabens Profile Interpretive Guide. Duluth, GA.

Niture SK, Refai L. Plant pectin: A potential source for cancer suppression. *American Journal of Pharmacology and Toxicology*. 2013;8(1):9-19.

Oxychlordane. TOXNET Toxicology Data Network. National Library of Medicine website. 2003. Accessed August 4, 2015. Available at: http://toxnet.nlm.nih.gov/cgi-bin/sis/search/a?dbs+hsdb:@term+@DOCNO+6771

Petriello MC, Newsome B, Hennig B. Influence of nutrition in PCB-induced vascular inflammation. *Environ Sci Pollut Res*. 2014;21:6410–6418.

Petrovska BB. Historical review of medicinal plants' usage. *Pharmacogn Rev*. 2012;6(11):1-5.

Rakel, David. *Integrative Medicine,* 3rd Edition. W.B. Saunders Company, 2012.

Rostami I, Juhasz AL. Assessment of persistent organic pollutant (POP) bioavailability and bioaccessibility for human health exposure assessment: A critical review. *Environmental Science and Technology.* 2011;41(7):623-656.

Schwalfenberg G, Genuis SJ, Rodushkin I. The benefits and risks of consuming brewed tea: beware of toxic element contamination. Hindawi Publishing Corporation. *Journal of Toxicology.* Volume 2013, Article ID 370460, 8 pages. **http://dx.doi.org/10.1155/2013/370460**

Sears ME, Genuis SJ. Environmental determinants of chronic disease and medical approaches: Recognition, avoidance, supportive therapy, and detoxification. *Journal of Environmental and Public Health.* Volume 2012, Article ID 356798, 15 pages. doi:10.1155/2012/356798

Sears ME. Chelation: Harnessing and enhancing heavy metal detoxification—A review. *The Scientific World Journal.* 2013, Article ID 219840, 13 pages **http://dx.doi.org/10.1155/2013/219840.**

Singh M, Sandhir R, Kiran R. Effects on antioxidant status of liver following atrazine exposure and its attenuation by vitamin E. *Experimental and Toxicologic Pathology.* 2011;63:269-276.

Volatile Solvents Guide. Metametrix Clinical Laboratory. Duluth, GA.

Yang M, Lee HS, Hwang MW, Jin M. Effects of Korean red ginseng (Panax Ginseng) on bisphenol A exposure and gynecologic complaints: single blind, randomized clinical trial of efficacy and safety. *BMC Complementary and Alternative Medicine.* 2014;14:265-274.

EPILOGUE

11 of the fastest growing green jobs. National Geographic website. 2016. Accessed April 7, 2016. Available at: **http://environment.nationalgeographic.com/environment/sustainable-earth/11-of-the-fastest-growing-green-jobs/#/rio-20-green-jobs-roof-top-garden_55050_600x450.jpg**

Bendig P, Maier L, Vetter W. Brominated vegetable oil in soft drinks – an underrated source of human organobromine intake. *Food Chemistry.* 2012;133:678–682.

Benford D, Bolger PM, Carthew P, Coulet M, DiNovi M, Leblanc JC, Renwick AG, Setzer W, Schlatter J, Smith B, Slob W, Williams G, Wildemann T. Application of the Margin of Exposure (MOE) approach to substances in food that are genotoxic and carcinogenic. *Food and Chemical Toxicology.* 2010;48:S2–S24.

Cogliano VJ, Baan R, Straif K, Grosse Y, Lauby-Secretan B, Ghissassi FE, Bouvard V, Benbrahim-Tallaa L, Guha N, Freeman C, Galichet L, Wild CP. Preventable exposures associated with human cancers. *J Natl Cancer Inst.* 2011;103:1827-1839.

Deribe E, Rosseland BO, Borgstrom R, Salbu B, Gebremariam Z, Dadebo E, Norli HR, Eklo OM. Bioaccumulation of persistent organic pollutants (POPs) in fish species from Lake Koka, Ethiopia: The influence of lipid content and trophic position. *Science of the Total Environment.* 2011;410-411:136–145.

DiGangi J, Schettler T, Cobbing M, Rossi M. Aggregate exposures to phthalates in humans. July 2002. Health Care Without Harm.

Genuis SJ. Fielding a current idea: exploring the public health impact of electromagnetic radiation. *Public Health.* 2008;122:113–124.

Genuis SJ. Nowhere to hide: Chemical toxicants and the unborn child. *Reproductive Toxicology.* 2009;28:115–116.

Genuis SJ. Toxicant Exposure and Mental Health—Individual, Social, and Public Health Considerations. *J Forensic Sci.* 2009;54(2):474-478.

Genuis SJ, Lipp CT. Electromagnetic hypersensitivity: Fact or fiction? *Science of the Total Environment.* 2012;414:103–112.

Genuis SJ, Schwalfenberg G, Siy A-KJ, Rodushkin I (2012) Toxic Element Contamination of Natural Health Products and Pharmaceutical Preparations. PLoS ONE 7(11): e49676.

doi:10.1371/journal.pone.0049676.

Haines DA, Murray J. Human biomonitoring of environmental chemicals—Early results of the 2007–2009 Canadian Health Measures Survey for males and females. *International Journal of Hygiene and Environmental Health.* 2012;215:133– 137.

Heinrich J. Influence of indoor factors in dwellings on the development of childhood asthma. *International Journal of Hygiene and Environmental Health.* 2011;214:1–25.

Mathew G, Unnikrishnan MK. The Emerging Environmental Burden from Pharmaceuticals. *Economic & Political Weekly.* 2012;18:31-35.

Montse M, Nadal M, Schuhmacher M, Domingo JL. Body burden monitoring of dioxins and other organic substances in workers at a hazardous waste incinerator. *International Journal of Hygiene and Environmental Health.* 2013;216:728-734.

Stoll ML. Green Chemistry Meets Green Business: A Match Long Overdue. *J Bus Ethics.* 2011;99:23–28.

Stuart M, Lapworth D, Crane E, Hart A. Review of risk from potential emerging contaminants in UK groundwater. *Science of the Total Environment.* 2012;416:1–21.

WHO Geneva 2002. Evaluation of certain food additives and contaminants. Fifty-seventh report of the Joint FAO/WHO Expert Committee on Food Additives – Carrageenan.

Yang X, Flowers RC, Weinberg HS, Singer PC. Occurrence and removal of pharmaceuticals and personal care products (PPCPs) in an advanced wastewater reclamation plant. *Water Research.* 2011;45:5218-5228.

CPSIA information can be obtained
at www.ICGtesting.com
Printed in the USA
BVHW060618010421
603820BV00002B/19

9 781732 704961